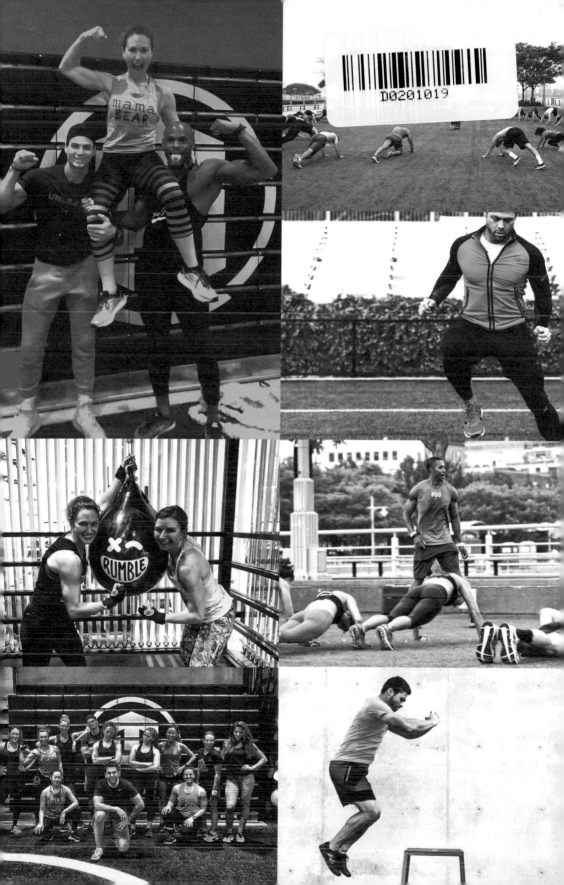

Becoming AGE LESS

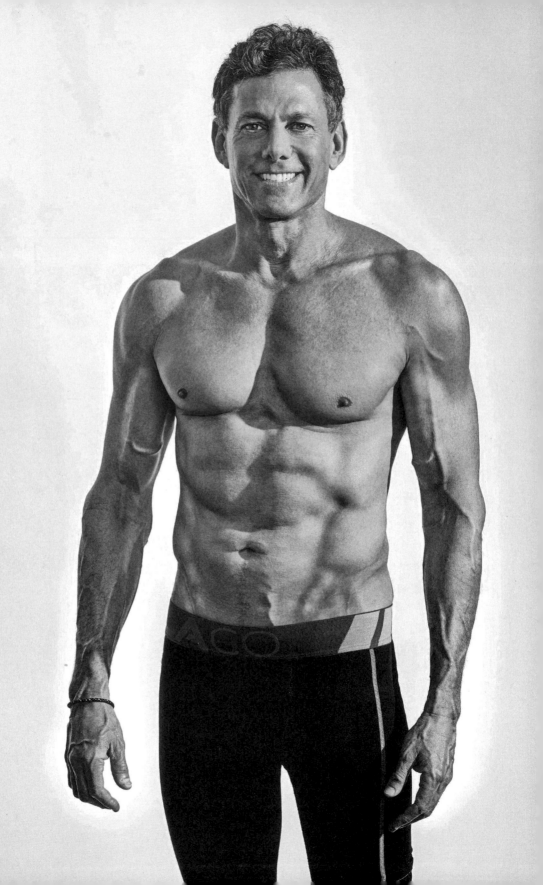

Becoming AGE LESS

The Four Secrets to Looking and Feeling Younger Than Ever

STRAUSS ZELNICK

with Zack Zeigler

This book proposes a program of diet and exercise recommendations for the reader to follow. However, you should consider a qualified medical professional (and, if you are pregnant, your ob-gyn) before starting this or any other fitness program. Please see your doctor's advice before making any decisions that affect your health or extreme changes in your diet, particularly if you suffer from any medical condition or have any symptom that may require treatment. As with any diet or exercise program, if at any time you experience discomfort, stop immediately and consult your physician.

Published in the United States by Galvanized Media and distributed by Simon & Schuster

Hardcover ISBN: 9781940358178

eBook ISBN: 9781940358192

Photographs by Brad Trent

simonandschuster.com

First edition

Book design by Joe Heroun

In memory of
the incredibly talented,
kind, and fit

SHAWN PERINE

CONTENTS

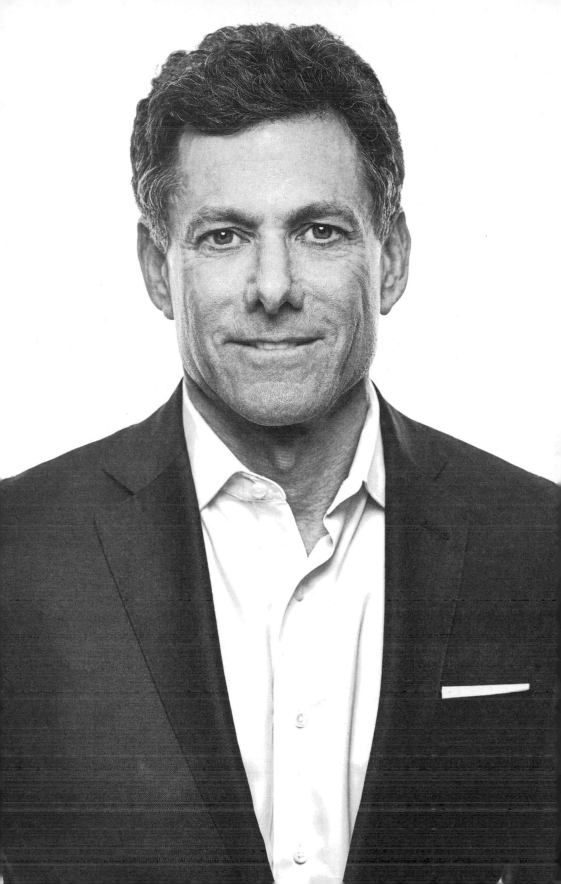

Foreword

LEGEND HAS IT that a reporter once asked Albert Einstein what man's greatest invention was, and the scientist, after a long pause, didn't respond with any of the usual answers, such as the wheel, the printing press, or even the theory of relativity. Instead, the man who forever changed our understanding of the universe simply replied: "Compound interest." Whether or not he actually uttered those words, I'd argue that compounding—the idea of something gaining value exponentially into the future through better decisions made in the present—is one of the greatest lessons any human being can ever learn. But I'm not talking about your 401(k). I'm talking about your health.

Most people know that genes play a dominant role in living longer, but that's only part of the equation. After all, for those of us not genetically bequeathed with magic genes ensuring we become centenarians—or even ensuring that we're fit, active, and looking great well into our sixth, seventh, and eighth decades—what can we do?

The answer is actually less about the exact details of *what* you should do and more about the mind-set of *how* you do it. And in *Becoming Ageless*, Strauss Zelnick, a man who is undeniably healthy and vibrant—who has built a body over time that appears truly to defy age—makes a compelling case for the following answer: Day in and day out, if you want to live longer and live better, you need a clear and basic understanding that the outcome of your journey is the sum of its steps.

Strauss is not just my patient. He's a dear friend, and our friendship has offered me a front-row seat to the discipline at the heart of his success. He is not in any way genetically superior to you. His greatest talent, at least when it comes to his health, is his capacity for consistency and the common sense with which he approaches all the health-minded topics you'll find in this book. Strauss knows there's a fine line between skipping a workout because you're busy and skipping one because your body needs a day off. He knows there's a fine line between indulging in a decadent dessert every once in a while and inhaling junk food because it's there and you're hungry. The challenge is discovering that line for yourself and walking it every day. And once you've discovered it, you can exploit the miracle of compounding your health.

There are no guarantees with your health, just as there are no guarantees with your wealth. As an entertainment-world executive at the top of his game for nearly four decades, Strauss knows this more than anyone. But he also knows that you can stack the odds in your favor by making sacrifices today that are worth the gains in the long term. And with the principles that he explains in *Becoming Ageless*, you'll be living longer—and with greater clarity of thought, mobility, and freedom from pain.

Ultimately, I hope that you take both Strauss's tactical insights about daily living *and* his strategic insight into the larger quest to live longer and better. After all, Strauss is living proof that if you're willing to consistently and incrementally implement small changes—while keeping your eye on the larger goal at all times—you'll boost your chances of living longer and living happier than you ever imagined.

Peter Attia, MD
FOUNDER, ATTIA MEDICAL, PC
NEW YORK, NY; SAN DIEGO, CA

Introduction

THE RIGHT QUESTION

TAKE A MOMENT and imagine yourself in old age.

Whether that's 10, 20, or even 50 years down the road from now, think hard and conjure an image of yourself in the twilight of your life.

What do you see?

If I had to guess, you're probably not thrilled by what immediately comes to mind. At best, maybe you're slower, grayer, and weaker—a shadow of your former self. At worst, you're so frail that everyday activities like lifting yourself out of a chair have become Herculean tasks.

Now clear that image from your mind.

Next, I'm going to ask you to repeat the exercise, except this time I'd like you to imagine yourself to be fitter, sharper, and more energized than you are right now.

I realize that sounds far-fetched, but I'd like you to picture it: There you are, in your 60s, 70s, or even your 80s. Sure, the signs of age are all there—your hair has thinned, your face has more wrinkles than before, and your step isn't *quite* as springy—but there are no wheelchairs, canes, or retirement homes in this future. And you're not passing the time confined to a Barcalounger or playing shuffleboard, either. If you're a tennis player, you're still storming the net with tenacity. If you're a runner, you're still attacking your neighborhood trails. If you are a boot-camp addict—as I am—you're still high-fiving your buddies in the park after a satisfying, sweat-soaked training session. Whatever it is you love doing, you're doing it with the energy of someone half your age, and your body isn't standing in your way.

Now, this is the part where I tell you that *this version* can become a reality, and that with the principles and lessons contained in *Becoming Ageless*, you can actually be in the best shape of your life at any age.

How do I know this?

Because I am living, breathing proof.

Right now I'm measurably fitter than I was 10 years ago. Fast-forward 12 months from now—when I'm 61 years old—and I intend to be in even *better* physical and mental condition than I am today. If you believe my fitness buddies, I have a body that's aging in reverse. Judge for yourself—the photographs in this book are recent and have not been retouched. I'm 6 feet and 160 pounds, with about 8 percent body fat. I train with former professional and college athletes in their 20s, 30s, and 40s, and I'm in the middle of the pack. And no, I'm not a certified trainer, exercise physiologist, nutritionist, or doctor. And no, I haven't spent my life competing in team sports or Ironmans. Frankly, I've never really considered myself an athlete at all.

What I am is a father, a husband, and a businessman, the CEO of Take-Two Interactive Software—the company behind blockbuster video games including *Grand Theft Auto* and *NBA 2K*—and a partner at Zelnick Media Capital (ZMC), a leading private equity firm based in New York City. Earlier in my career, I ran the film studio 20th Century Fox and later became CEO of the global music company BMG Entertainment. Now,

I'm not reeling off my résumé just to stoke my own sense of self-satisfaction. I'm just telling you who I am, which is a hardworking, passionate guy who is living a full life by embracing the power of consistency and daily determination in achieving goals—whatever those goals may be.

Four mornings a week, I bolt out of bed to train with The Program, a group of like-minded fitness enthusiasts in New York City who have dedicated themselves to pursuing healthy, strong, and productive lives. (You'll see photos of many at the beginning and end of this book.) We have about 80 members total, with roughly 15 to 20 participating in a given workout. From boot camp to hot power yoga to weight training and spinning, our 6 a.m. training routines vary by the day, but what remains constant is our encouragement and drive to present our best selves both in and out of the gym. Believe it or not, three or four days a week, I will actually head back to the gym for a post-work workout. I know that's a lot of exercise, but I love to train, and over time I've managed to work my body up to that level of physical activity—and I firmly believe that, if that's something you'd like to accomplish, you can, too.

The Program has become more than a workout group to me. It's a movement that plays a hugely important role in my life. Throughout *Becoming Ageless*, you'll hear firsthand from several of my team members—people of all ages and body types—who have experienced positive changes through their involvement. As I'll explain later, you don't need The Program to unlock your best self. But *Becoming Ageless* is filled with countless useful tips and unique principles you'd find if you *did* train with The Program. And, as you'll soon discover, there are a lot of great exercise routines in this book straight from Rafique "Flex" Cabral, one of The Program's top trainers.

However, before you hit the gym and set yourself on the path to a *Becoming Ageless* body, first ask yourself a question— a different question. Because I believe most of us begin too many things in life by asking the wrong one: We tend to ask, "How?"

As in, *How do I lose weight? How do I earn a promotion? How do I get in shape? How do I afford a new car? How can I feel better about myself? How do I stay young and healthy?*

Asking *how* you're going to achieve a dietary, fitness, material, or spiritual goal is unlikely to yield the result you seek. Instead, start by asking yourself a far more important question. It's one I asked myself years ago: "What do I want?"

That answer will drive every decision you make. It will also make the *how* easier to pinpoint and, eventually, accomplish.

This is how I answered my question:

I know I want to . . .

◆ **Live as long and healthily as possible while being cogent and mobile.**

◆ **Be fit and strong.**

◆ **Perform my job at my highest level.**

◆ **Have warm and meaningful relationships with my family and friends.**

◆ **Push my limits both mentally and physically.**

◆ **Look good in and out of clothes.**

◆ **Feel youthful, happy, satisfied, and as stress-free as possible.**

◆ **Be spiritually connected.**

◆ **Help others achieve their goals.**

What I don't want (and I assume you don't, either) is to be limited or defined by my age. Yet sometimes, we forget that, while there's no stopping the passage of time, we can control how well we age. Because the notion that you'll get too old to run marathons, too weak for century rides, too fragile to ski or snowboard, or too fatigued to keep up with your grandchildren at a park is just plain wrong. It doesn't matter if you're a millennial or a centenarian: Right now, you have all the resources you need to make changes to obtain or reclaim the life you want. That's if you know what you want.

So think about what you want. Be honest and don't edit your thoughts. Contemplate it for a week if you need to. Then write down five to 10 goals. Write them right here in this book:

1. _____

2. _____

3. _____

4. _____

5. _____

6. _____

7. _____

8. _____

9. _____

10. _____

For those who want to recalibrate their lives, I want this book to provide support and advice—especially when it comes to reaping the benefits of a life steeped in strength, fitness, and health.

You can attain and maintain a full life with a lot less effort than you think. But let's be clear: There are no shortcuts. I know that contradicts what's marketed to you by the health and fitness industry:

- ◆ **Washboard Abs in 12 Days!**
- ◆ **A Slimmer You in 3 Easy Moves!**
- ◆ **A New Body Tomorrow!**

I started my career in sales at Columbia Pictures, so I understand the marketing strategy behind such compelling—although unrealistic—promises. But what actually works is the opposite of a quick fix. No transformation can be achieved overnight. If I had tried to do too much, too fast, and ramped up my training from three workouts a week to 12 without preparing my body and mind, I wouldn't have succeeded. In fact, I would've injured myself. Instead, the *Becoming Ageless* method is ultimately a smarter, gentler, and far more sustainable one that will ease you into a new way of living—and keep you there.

I'm not making this up. Over the past decade, I've immersed myself in the science and practice of healthy eating and exercise, and today, it's not uncommon for people to ask me as many questions about fitness, health, and nutrition as they do about business and investing. Everything I've learned about living a healthy, active life I've included in this book to share with you.

Being fit means different things to different people, and it changes at different stages of our lives. As we get older, strength and fitness become even more important, not only for health, but also for having the continued energy and stamina to stay competitive and productive in our careers. Strength and fitness—and the side benefit of stress reduction—are critical to helping you get the most enjoyment out of your passions and your relationships with others. I hope that this book helps you recognize all the good that can come from getting back in shape, and that it inspires you to use its practical lessons and advice to become "ageless."

Once you've adopted healthier eating habits and a consistent fitness routine and feel mentally and spiritually stronger, I'm going to ask you to stick with the *Becoming Ageless* plan for 12 weeks. Solidifying those habits over 90 days will require modest adjustments, sacrifices, and effort. But the plan is specifically set up to offer you enough time to find the best way to adjust to your new training and nutrition plans, work them harmoniously into your schedule, and make them permanent.

Now, if you feel like you're too old, too weak, too out of shape, too lazy, or too out of touch with the fast-paced world of fitness trends to unlock your best body, I'm here to tell you that you're flat-out wrong.

How do I know this?

Experience.

"Honey, you really don't look all that good…"

I GREW UP IN Boston and outside New York City in the late 1970s, when gyms weren't as ubiquitous as they are now and weight lifting was exclusively for beefy football players and a select group of bodybuilders. My father was an intellectual and a lawyer. He was a gentle and modest man, but not the type of guy who'd want to play catch. Together with my mom—the disciplinarian—my parents sought to raise my five siblings and me as sophisticated, cultured, and well-mannered children. As a result, sports—especially contact sports—were not part of the equation. Tennis and swimming were permitted, as was riding horses. But above all, I enjoyed reading. I would tear through everything from Hardy Boys adventures to adult-oriented tomes such as *Manchild in the Promised Land*, an autobiographical novel about an inner-city kid from Harlem who ends up in reform school, with rabid enthusiasm.

I took up running in high school and squash in graduate school—which was also the first time I ever tried strength training. My initial bare-bones strength routine consisted of 10-minute sessions of push-ups, pull-ups, and sit-ups. Next I tried the newfangled trend of "state-of-the-art" Nautilus equipment, the selling point being that it better maintained tension and resistance throughout an exercise and was therefore more efficient at full-body training. Who wouldn't want that?

Turns out, *I* didn't want that.

All I could do to get through the workout was to remind myself of how good a shower would feel afterward. Besides, my primary interest wasn't my body. It was my work.

In 1980, I was hired by Columbia Pictures to be the director of international television sales. I had no business experience to speak of, and it was at least two levels above where I should have been hired. But I was fortunate they took a chance on me right out of school, and even more fortunate when they promoted me to vice president of international television sales early on. I eventually left Columbia in 1986 to join Vestron Pictures, a rapidly growing independent film company, where the first movie I green-lit was *Dirty Dancing*, which became for many years the highest-grossing independent movie of all time.

By then I was 30 years old, driven, and passionate about my work as president of a film studio. I soon met my future wife, Wendy Belzberg, on a blind date, and I knew immediately she was the one. (Suffice it to say, that feeling wasn't mutual. She hated my haircut. And how I was dressed. But she saw enough in me to agree to another date, which led to another—and another—and, later, a marriage and three amazing children.) Through it all, despite training three days a week, my health was not a huge priority in my life.

By the mid-'90s, I'd been an executive for more than a decade. Because I had never gained weight, proper nutrition wasn't of great concern to me. My meals were often big and heavy on carbs and sweets. Although I didn't necessarily look out of shape, I didn't look or feel my best, either. This was about the time that I read *Younger Next Year*, the hit book by Chris Crowley and Henry S. Lodge, which was a general health and wellness guide for people ages 60 and up. Even though I was 38 and hitting the gym three times a week, it resonated with me. It taught me that if I wanted to live a good life, I needed to eat a moderate diet and work out six days a week. Yet I still lacked the motivation to make the necessary changes. Then one day, I returned home from the gym—my workout clothes lacking any visible trace of sweat—and my wife cracked a joke: "Honey, you really don't look all that good for a guy who spends so much time in the gym."

Bam! That did it.

My first step was to get a trainer. I began working out with Jeong Kim three mornings a week at 6 a.m. Kim is a former Olympic water polo player, and he put me through the paces with challenging moves and strict form. I learned about the role methodical resistance training plays in transforming the body.

By my 40s, I started to diversify my fitness—boxing, yoga, and other high-intensity exercises were added into the mix. I also finally began to address my poor diet. I cut out alcohol and all of the greasy dishes I used to consume without thinking twice. In my 50s, I was determined to build more muscle and get my body fat well below the 10 percent mark—a must in order to reveal defined abs. So I mapped out a plan that would get me the body I wanted and began to execute it. I did my home-work, surrounded myself with positive, knowledgeable people, and then went about fulfilling the answer to the question that started it all: What do I want?

Eventually, this led to the creation of The Program.

The Program

ABOUT SIX YEARS ago, a few fitness buddies and I unofficially launched The Program. It was more than a decade in the making, and in its infancy was a guys-only morning cycling group that morphed into a coed team of 80 or so members of different ages and backgrounds. We train together in New York City four days a week at 6 a.m. in pursuit of healthy, strong, and productive lives. We're connected by the spirit that comes from setting and achieving goals, being healthy, building strength, and finding joy in pushing ourselves beyond where we originally believed were our physical and mental limits.

What truly makes The Program special, though, isn't the exercises we do or the variety in our weekly training; it's the fact that we're a tribe of friendly, upbeat people who share a common goal and encourage one another to succeed. We are mutually supportive despite our vast differences in upbringing, fitness levels, and age. The Program didn't appear overnight— it was something that evolved organically over time into something with deeper connections than any single workout partner could provide. In fitness, there is little that can substitute for the power of the group dynamic. When you share effort, struggle, and sweat, you create something far greater than a calorie burn. You create an energy, an intensity, a sense of accountability, a spirit of teamwork, and an aura that can carry you not only through a grueling workout, but also through many of life's obstacles. Above all, over and over, The Program has demonstrated how the unity created from a group whose members share a communal goal can, without fail, uplift the team both physically and emotionally.

When people ask me how to create something like The Program, I tell them to find people to train with—friends, clients, strangers, anyone they enjoy spending time with who wants to train. Instead of setting up a business meeting over cocktails or meeting a friend for pizza, suggest a workout. Once you develop that habit, in time, you'll build a network.

As you read *Becoming Ageless*, you will learn to structure your life in ways that encourage consistency and a commitment to fitness. For instance, the night before I hit the gym I prepack my gym bag for the sake of efficiency; I sleep with my phone in a room adjacent to my bedroom to ensure I get out of bed when its alarm sounds; and I keep my espresso machine in my bathroom closet—far from my bedroom—ready to brew. Why do I keep an espresso machine in a closet instead of in my kitchen? Because my wife of 27 years, Wendy, has on more than one occasion voiced displeasure at my early-morning commotion—gentle alarm tones and the machine's faint whirring included—which wakes her up.

But don't worry. I'm not asking you to wake up at dawn or trying to recruit you into The Program. I use The Program only as an example of one way to achieve fitness goals and to make the point that it's easier and more fun to work toward any goal with friends as opposed to alone.

Above all, I want you to know that developing the body and life you want isn't about achieving perfection in a few weeks. It isn't about diving into the deep end of the pool. It's about putting a toe in the water, then a foot, then a knee, then a leg, and so on. The way to change—and to sustain that change—is to take your time. Be gentle on your body, and your body will respond by wanting to do more.

That is the key to success.

Best of all, it doesn't have to take decades to figure it out. With a gentle approach, you will start feeling changes almost immediately and seeing modest improvement within as few as three weeks. Those early results will encourage motivation. Before you know it, 90 days will have gone by and you will have lost weight, gained muscle, and begun to see dramatic differences between the old you and the new you. What's more, you will feel remarkably better mentally as well as physically.

What follows in the subsequent pages is *how*—not only how to get fitter, but also how to do so while living in a rewarding, satisfying, and balanced way. For me, these are the four key elements to a good life—to an ageless life:

- ◆ **Fitness**
- ◆ **Nutrition**
- ◆ **Health**
- ◆ **Soul**

They are the four pillars of this book. In each section, I will highlight systems that will work for you in your own pursuit of fitness, physical and mental strength, and a healthier life. These are grounded not only in my experience, but also in academic research. The formula isn't complex. It's about teaching yourself how to make better, sustainable choices that can ultimately be woven into your lifestyle. This book is about how the people around me and I reshaped our bodies and our lives.

Ultimately, I hope that you get more from *Becoming Ageless* than just step-by-step instructions for executing a burpee (which is on page 237, in case that is of interest), why you should vary your workouts, and how to make nutritious food delicious. The ideal takeaway would be an understanding that building physical, mental, and spiritual strength will improve just about everything—from family life and friendships to business success and self-confidence.

You'll see that you absolutely can get what you want—with no expiration date.

THE PROGRAM: CORE VALUES

We are inclusive but selective. The Program is an inviting group of athletes who support one another in pursuit of improving ourselves and those around us.

We strive to inspire those around us by showing the camaraderie, energy, and results that come from being a part of our lifestyle.

Each individual is accountable to and responsible for the team and must be willing to make sacrifices for change.

We document our journey to recognize and celebrate individual and team growth. We appreciate the efforts of others and commend those who break personal, fitness, and professional barriers.

We unselfishly share our love of fitness, health, and The Program, asking for nothing in return.

It's not just about fitness: Our relationship may start in the weight room, at the studio, or on a bike, but our attitude extends to the way we treat one another, ourselves, and those we encounter every day.

THE *BECOMING AGELESS* PLAN

This is the definitive 12-week plan for those who aspire to look, feel, and perform at their peak—regardless of age, fitness level, or athletic ability. This plan forgoes a rigid cold-turkey approach for one that encourages making small yet effective changes that focus on the four pillars of youthful living and can help you both figuratively and literally age in reverse. In other words, you won't deal with any inflexible diets or unrealistic workout demands. *Becoming Ageless* instead features peer-reviewed studies, personal experience, and many success stories that demonstrate how a gentle but calculated approach to building a healthier mind and body not only promotes vitality, a youthful appearance, and self-confidence, but also opens the door to sustaining deeper connections with friends and loved ones.

You'll Eat

Three meals per day from the unlimited and limited categories (see page 94)—with a focus on more fibrous and protein-centric foods.

Figure out your caloric needs by multiplying your goal weight by 12. (So a person aiming to weigh 180 pounds should plan to consume around 2,160 calories each day.)

You'll Drink

At least 16 more ounces of water per day than you did before reading this book. You'll choose from unlimited, limited, and highly restricted drinks (see page 93).

You'll Reduce

Added sugar and soda intake meaningfully.

You'll Work Out

This plan (see page 210) is designed to make physical activity a fixture in your everyday life, beginning with 2 weeks of body-weight exercises, walking, and stretching.

By Week 3, you'll perform your first strength circuit—1 round, 9 exercises, 5 to 10 reps for each.

By Week 12, you will have eased into doing 3 weekly training sessions that consist of 3 sets of 12 reps per exercise or 3–5 sets of 5 reps, for a total of 45 minutes to 1 hour per session.

You'll Connect

Every day you're encouraged to spend at least 3 to 5 minutes on any of these:

- Prayer (group or individual)
- Meditation
- Deep breathing
- Yoga

Your Diagnostics

IN THE BUSINESS world, they call it "benchmarking."

It's the standard practice of taking stock of your company's performance—analyzing reams of data on what's working, seeing what's not working, and comparing your metrics with those of your competitors—so you can make better, more informed decisions as you navigate your organization down the road to success. Yes, this is "Management 101" (if not "Common Sense 101"), but you'd be amazed at how few companies go through the process of giving themselves regular checkups as they're planning their long-term strategies. Pretty dumb, right? If you're running a Fortune 500 business and you don't know your strengths and weaknesses today, how could you possibly build a stronger, healthier, and more vibrant company tomorrow?

Now, I hate to put you on the spot, but I have a few questions: Have you ever had a prostate screening? A mammogram? When was the last time you had your blood pressure checked? Or simply stepped on a scale and weighed yourself?

It should go without saying that if you want to live a longer, richer, fuller life, it's absolutely imperative that you take stock of your health right now.

There are countless excuses that people use to avoid medical checkups—a hatred of needles, the expense, and the time commitment are a few. However, the most common might be the fear of receiving unfavorable test results. A downside to this approach is that ailments that go undetected or without treatment cannot be addressed, cured, or managed. Health diagnostics are, after all, more about *prevention* than detection. Consider these statistics from a survey conducted by the Commonwealth Fund:

> **"Fitness, nutrition, health, and soul are the four pillars of this book."**

- Half of the male respondents had not had a physical exam or cholesterol test in the prior 12 months.

- 41 percent of men age 50 and older had not been screened for prostate cancer in the previous 12 months; 60 percent had not been screened for colon cancer. These deadly diseases are highly curable, but only if detected early.

- 25 percent of men admitted to waiting as long as possible before seeking medical help.

Yes, that's a lot of people out there not checking their benchmarks. In my case, along with standard checkups—a yearly physical, eye and skin exams, dental cleanings every six months, and standard cancer-prevention procedures such as chest X rays and colonoscopies—I have my blood checked every three months to monitor how my body is reacting to my diet and exercise routine by my doctor, nutrition scientist Peter Attia, MD, one of our most brilliant thinkers about food and longevity. That's more frequently than most people would need or want a blood test, but I enjoy tracking and analyzing.

If you've accepted the premise of this book—that you can make meaningful, beneficial changes systematically in incremental ways to improve your quality of life—you can also commit to taking age-appropriate tests and having regular checkups. Even if you're not in the shape that you want—*especially* if you're not in the shape that you want—you need to know where you are to figure out where you're going and how to get there.

That starts by scheduling a physical. Along with asking your doctor which tests you should have based on your age and family history, plan to cover the following: cholesterol (HDL and LDL), triglycerides, glucose, insulin, hemoglobin A1C, complete blood count, CRP, and homocysteine. For men, add testosterone, DHEA, and PSA to that list.

However, the most important thing you can do is get screened for common, curable cancers. Many cancers show no visible symptoms until they grow and/or spread. But early detection—in areas such as the colon or prostate—can allow a doctor to eradicate the disease. Harvard University researchers tracked nearly 89,000 adults for 22 years and found that men who had a colonoscopy or sigmoidoscopy were, on the whole, 56 percent less likely to develop colon cancer than those not screened.

On the following page I've included all the major areas that you should have checked by a professional. And once you know where you stand, you can take your first step forward.

A Beginner's Guide to Regular Checkups

THE CHART AT right will help you navigate your appointments. Guidelines in this first chart are based on U.S. government recommendations; refer to your primary doctor regarding specific follow-ups.

PHYSICIAN'S CHECKUP LIST

Annual unless otherwise noted.

	In Your 30s	In Your 40s	In Your 50s
Physical	X	X	X
Blood Test Including cholesterol and blood sugar	X	X	X
Sexually Transmitted Diseases	X	X	X
Dental Exam and Cleaning Every 6 months	X	X	X
Eye Exam	X	X	X
Skin Screening	X	X	X
Colorectal Cancer Screenings Every 3 to 5 years over the age of 30	X	X	X
Prostate Cancer Screening	X	X	X
Osteoporosis Screening			X
Lung Cancer Screening (chest X ray)			X

A Beginner's Guide to Self-Examinations

THE LIST BELOW contains tests that can help monitor weight-loss efforts, screen for hypertension, and gauge fitness progression—no doctor's visit required.

SELF-TEST: RECOMMENDATIONS

WEIGHT

If you're trying to lose weight, weigh yourself once weekly on the same day and at the same time until you reach your target weight. If you are comfortable with your weight, use the mirror as your guide.

BLOOD PRESSURE

Check your blood pressure monthly, either with your own device or at a pharmacy or gym. Take it more often if you have high blood pressure.

BODY FAT

An immersion test is the only truly accurate measure, but a body-fat scale or caliper—even though they aren't always 100 percent accurate—will suffice for occasional checks. Watching the numbers drop can be a motivator or, if they've stalled, can serve as a reminder to revisit the question: What do you want?

PERFORMANCE

If you're able to achieve more physically than you were the previous month and you feel better while doing it, you've made progress. Compared with last month, can you do more push-ups? Can you run faster or for longer distances? Do you feel stronger during your workouts? The answers indicate that you are or are not making progress. Use these measures to keep pushing toward achieving your goals.

Part One

GET WITH THE PROGRAM

The ultimate exercise regimen
for getting lean, reducing stress,
and feeling energized—for life

I'VE BEEN FORTUNATE to be involved in several successful turnarounds in my business career. When I took over 20th Century Fox in 1989, the studio was last place in the market and putting out a meager six movies a year. A year later, we were No. 1 at the box office and went on to release more than 20 films a year for three straight years. On my first day at BMG Entertainment, in the mid-'90s, we were fifth out of six record companies in the marketplace. When I left, six years later, we were ranked second and posting record profits. And since founding ZMC, in 2000, my company has taken several companies that previously were losing money—Columbia Music Entertainment; Lillian Vernon; Time Life; and Take-Two Interactive, which ZMC controls—and turned them into valuable, profit-generating brands.

The approach I used to make these turnarounds didn't involve guesswork. Instead, we used a priority matrix.

Imagine a graph with four quadrants. Mark the y-axis "Impact" and the x-axis "Effort." When you want to turn around a business, the best way forward is first to employ strategies that you consider to be "low effort, high impact." After that, you may try strategies that are "high effort, high impact." The third and less ideal would be "low effort, low impact." But whatever you do, avoid anything that falls into the category of "high effort, low impact." The idea behind this is simple: When you want real, measurable results, you need a calculated, efficient, and promising path forward.

"Be gentle on your body, and your body will respond by wanting to do more."

When you start the *Becoming Ageless* workout and eating plans, you'll find that I've used the same approach for helping you achieve your health and wellness goals. And what goes into each box hinges on the list of wants I asked you to create

PRIORITY MATRIX

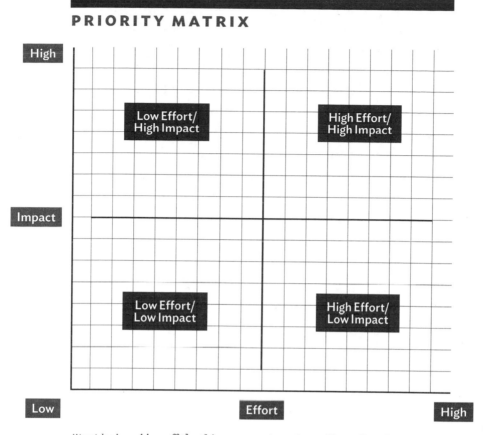

Start by knocking off the things you categorize as "low effort, high impact." Then take care of items that are "high effort, high impact," finally moving to the "low effort, low impact" section. Consider anything "high effort, low impact" as a misuse of your time and resources.

on page 16. But there is a good chance that your list of wants resembles mine, especially if you're fueled in part by vanity. After all, who doesn't want to be fit, strong, and healthy—and feel comfortable and look good in a bathing suit?

In that case, plan to usher in change slowly and be gentle with yourself by executing "low effort, high impact" actions first. Start by drinking more water (and less soda and alcohol), taking walks, exercising one or two times per week, eating an apple instead of a candy bar, and minimizing your consumption of food that comes in bags or boxes. "High effort, high impact" things, meanwhile, might be quitting smoking or stamping out added sugar from your diet.

But whatever your matrix looks like, exercise is essential, and strength training is especially important to your health and well-being. I would argue that it's as important as choosing not to smoke, wearing your seat belt when you drive, eating a balanced diet, and getting a good night's sleep.

If you want to stay fit, strong, and active, regular exercise is absolutely necessary—almost everything that declines physiologically as you get older will only improve with exercise.

I don't obsessively step on a scale or look in the mirror to gauge my body-fat percentage. I just love to train and have slowly worked up to seven to 12 workouts per week. Plus, my mind and body operate better when I follow a workout-heavy routine.

Your fitness goals will ultimately determine how often and how intensely you'll need to exercise to achieve success. And keep this in mind: You don't have to live in the gym. However, if you need more motivation to break a sweat on a consistent basis, here are some other benefits worth remembering:

Exercise Helps You Feel Younger

MUSCLE MASS STARTS to decline after age 30, and according to Harvard researchers, most men will lose about 30 percent of their muscle mass during their lifetimes. Engaging in progressive resistance training—using strength-building exercise to improve strength and endurance—can help preserve muscle mass. Research shows that fast-twitch muscle fibers—the ones responsible for generating power and explosive strength—shrink twice as fast as the slow-twitch fibers responsible for endurance. This is important because fast-twitch fibers help you perform explosive, athletic moves when you play sports. Later, when you're in your 90s, they are the ones that you'll rely on to help you get out of a chair or regain your balance quickly if you trip. If you target fast-twitch muscles with the proper strength and stretching exercises (like the ones shown in this book), you'll become a better athlete now and keep your muscle tone and ability to react quickly for decades to come.

Turn adversity into opportunity.

—Katie Sullivan, 28, The Program

In February 2013, a New York City cab traveling 30 mph hit Katie as she was crossing the street. Injuries to her face, shoulder, leg, meniscus, ACL, and MCL required 10 surgeries and left her wheelchair-bound for months, says Katie, a former lacrosse player at Colgate University. "Many doctors told me that being physically fit saved my life," she says.

Katie set incremental goals for recovery. The first was to walk again. She then said, "If I can walk, I can run." After she could run, the goal was to complete a half-marathon. Now she competes in triathlons.

As a member of The Program, Katie found support in her desire to improve her fitness. She even changed careers to work in the fitness industry. Our morning exercise has changed her life. "After a workout, I'm ready for the rest of the day. By 6:45 a.m., I'm feeling confident and accomplished, and I know I can take on whatever the rest of the day throws my way."

In fact, studies have shown that even in their 90s, people can physiologically turn back the clock after only a few weeks of regular weight-bearing exercise. This, in part, helps explain why I feel like I have the energy of a guy in his 20s, not his 60s.

Exercise Slows the Aging Process

A STUDY AT Brigham Young University determined that vigorous exercise had the ability to slow the aging of cells by nearly a decade in men and women. Researchers analyzed more than 6,000 subjects and found that high levels of exercise—running 30 to 40 minutes per day for at least five days per week—helped preserve telomere length. Telomeres are protein caps on the ends of chromosomes; shorter telomeres have been linked to an increase in age-related diseases, including cancer and stroke.

Exercise Supports Longevity

NO ONE KNOWS how long he or she will live, but there's something you can do to dramatically improve your chances of living longer: aerobic exercise. A Stanford University School of Medicine study on the effects running has on aging tracked 538 runners over age 50 and compared them with a similar group of non-runners. Nineteen years after the study began, only 15 percent of the runners had died, compared with 34 percent of the non-runners. The study also determined that runners had fewer disabilities and a much longer span of time when they could enjoy an active life. In other words: Make a habit of breaking a sweat every day.

Exercise Boosts Cognitive Abilities

WHEN YOU EXERCISE vigorously, you flood your brain with a greater supply of blood, which can keep your gray matter healthy and growing (a process called neurogenesis). The journal *Neurology* published a study suggesting that exercise helped keep the mind sharp and slowed down brain decline by 10 years. In the study, seniors who exercised regularly at moderate to intense levels were found to have retained more mental skills over the next five years than the seniors who did light exercise.

Additional research concluded that exercise improves the executive function of our brains—that is, the ability to do complex tasks, remember a series of numbers, think abstractly, and plan for future events. A meta-analysis of 18 studies found that people between the ages 55 and 80 who exercised regularly for 30 to 45 minutes per session outperformed non-exercisers by four times on tests of executive function.

Exercise Improves Mood

YOU ALMOST ALWAYS feel better, happier, and more confident after a workout. Aerobic exercise, in particular, has been shown to alleviate anxiety, stress, and even the frustrations around focus for people with attention deficit disorder. One landmark study at the University of Texas Southwestern demonstrated just how powerful exercise can be for mental health. In the study, 80 people suffering from depression were placed into one of five groups. Two of the groups did moderately intense aerobics for 30 minutes three to five days a week. Two other groups did low-intensity aerobics. And a fifth group did only stretches. After 12 weeks, those who worked out intensely three to five days a week reduced their depressive symptoms by nearly 50 percent, an effect equal to what would be expected from a prescription antidepressant medication. The UT Southwestern researchers pointed out that the effects were best when the exercise was rigorous and was sustained for at least 30 minutes.

Exercise Builds Stronger Bones

NOT ONLY DO you lose muscle mass as you age, but you also lose bone mass—even in your spine. When that happens, you can develop rounded shoulders and a hunched back, making you look much older. Fortunately, strength training can reverse bone loss. In one study reported in the *Journal of Applied Physiology*, subjects who performed 16 weeks of weight training boosted their hip bone density and increased blood levels—a marker of bone growth—by 19 percent.

Exercise Improves Insulin Sensitivity

THE HORMONE INSULIN is the key that unlocks our cells so that glucose, our body's main source of food, can enter and be used for energy. The problem is, when we constantly eat sugary, carbohydrate-rich foods that raise our blood sugar, our bodies must release more and more insulin to deal with it. Over time, our cells can become resistant to insulin, blood sugar may continue to rise, and type 2 diabetes may ultimately result. The good news is that regular exercise can actually reverse insulin resistance even if you don't change your diet. In fact, a single intense exercise session can increase insulin sensitivity for more than 16 hours, improving blood sugar control.

You can find many more science-backed reasons for why you should engage in regular exercise, but probably the most important reason is the way exercise will make your body and mind feel. It's what motivates me every day.

In this section, I'll also explain my research-based fitness practices and why each is so important to my overall approach. Taken together, my workouts include the following five elements that yield a dynamic, athletic, lean, and strong body—an ageless body:

Fitness is the journey.

—Jay Hass, 55, The Program

J ay didn't consider himself a jock growing up, but he does now. In high school he played varsity soccer but wasn't the star of the team. His mom introduced him to running—and it stuck. At 17, he completed his first marathon. Now in his 50s, he's still a runner. He once ran 10 miles in just over an hour and finished a 5K at a 5:42-mile pace. He insists on being in the top 5 percent overall of any race he enters, no matter his age, and he wants to win his age group. To date, Jay has run 22 marathons, including the Boston Marathon five times. He does some strength training and stretching, but his passion is being out on the road. In fact, he has run some 31,000 miles outdoors but has run on a treadmill only seven times in his life.

"The inherent nature of fitness is the journey. It's the sights I've seen: the urban alleys and seaside pathways I've explored by accident, the squinty sunsets and shivering sunrises, the view from Teton Pass at 8,800 feet and the rutted chalky basin of Death Valley, the snow freezing my eyelashes," he says. "Low-fiving smiling kids in wheelchairs along the Boston Marathon course, inspired to the point of tears. Today, I paid some bills and was going to put them in the mailbox outside. Then I looked at the clock. The post office was closing in 30 minutes. It's four miles away. So I ran there instead. That, to me, is the joy of being fit—the journey. And the gratitude that I feel every day for being able to take the journey."

1) Strength

I HAVE GOOD friends who run—and only run—and it's great that they find enjoyment in that activity. For holistic health and lifelong fitness, however, you need to incorporate some kind of strength training. Building lean muscle helps not only to increase metabolism, but also to fortify your body to handle everything life throws at you throughout any given day.

Remember the decrepit and much-worse-off version of yourself that you initially imagined? Unfortunately, that becomes a reality for many people in their 70s and 80s; they experience difficulty walking or even getting out of bed because they've lost muscle and strength in their legs. But the process starts much earlier. After age 30, your muscle mass naturally declines by roughly 3 to 5 percent per decade if you don't exercise. That may not seem like a lot, but it adds up. And remember that skeletal muscle consumes a few more calories per day than fat, so having less of it means fewer calories burned and more stored as fat.

2) Balance

YOUR BODY ALSO needs to know that it can move in all directions and support itself in unpredictable and athletic movements. That's why I incorporate flexibility training into my routines—stretching muscles and getting into different positions help me reduce the risk of injury and support all my other styles of training.

3) Intensity

I DON'T BOTHER just going through the motions. Why waste time? Almost all my training sessions are high-intensity—not only because of the efficiency in burning calories during the workout and the metabolic effects of burning calories after intense exercise, but also because the intensity leads to higher energy throughout the day. What is an intense workout? I define it as training with minimal rest periods—that means no sitting around texting or chatting with friends between sets. After a light warm-up you push yourself—hard. Rest as needed, but then go hard again until the final rep.

High-intensity workouts are both efficient and effective. And one particular kind of intense workout protocol, called high-intensity interval training, or HIIT for short, is among the best. HIIT workouts mix periods of all-out effort with short periods of recovery and can be done with various aerobic activities:

- ◆ **Walking**
- ◆ **Running**
- ◆ **Stair climbing**
- ◆ **Cycling**
- ◆ **Rowing**
- ◆ **Cross-country skiing**
- ◆ **Swimming**
- ◆ **Body-weight exercises**

You can even incorporate HIIT techniques into your weight-training routine.

In a recent study, researchers monitored two groups of exercisers—one that performed steady-state cardio (like running at a consistent pace) for 30 minutes three times a week and another that did 20 minutes of HIIT exercise three times a week. The high-intensity exercisers lost 2 percent of their body fat and gained two pounds of muscle; the steady-state exercisers lost virtually no body fat, but did drop one pound.

Other research published in the *Journal of Obesity* showed that HIIT exercisers reduced substantial belly fat while increasing lean muscle mass and aerobic power.

4) Variety

DOING THE SAME workout routine every day, every week, every year, for most of us, gets old fast. Boring workouts lead to missed workouts. Avoid falling into that trap by challenging your body in multiple ways to promote continual progress and to keep monotony at bay.

5) Community

I RARELY TRAIN alone. When I train with The Program, we encourage and coach one another to perform better to help each member realize that we're capable of doing more than we ever thought we could. It's why in any fitness regimen you choose to participate in, I encourage you to make other people part of it.

CHAPTER 1

Unlock Your Inner Strength

No matter your body type, acquiring more muscle is the foundation for an ageless body that performs as good as it looks.

THE FOUNDATION FOR a successful business is made up of its values, culture, goals, plans, and people. The foundation for your home is a concrete block. The foundation for a healthy meal is a robust piece of protein and fresh vegetables. The foundation for meeting and greeting someone is a firm handshake, eye contact, and a smile. In any aspect of life, the foundation is what dictates your approach, your growth, and your success. With a sturdy foundation, there are no limits. With a weak or shaky foundation, there is no future.

When I'm running a business, my job is to attract, motivate, and retain the most creative and passionate people in the industry to build a team that breeds success. In other words, the team is the foundation.

When I green-lit my first film, *Dirty Dancing*, it went on to become the highest-grossing independent film of all time. But I can't and won't take credit for its success. I was a *part* of its success, but the effort was collaborative and relied on scores of talented people pursuing their passion.

At Fox we produced blockbusters like *Home Alone, Sleeping with the Enemy, Die Hard 2,* and *The Abyss.* During my tenure at BMG, we released records by Toni Braxton, Backstreet Boys, Notorious B.I.G., and Whitney Houston, among others. In the video game industry, we've had runaway success with titles like *Grand Theft Auto, NBA 2K, Borderlands, Red Dead Redemption,* and *Civilization.* In every case, the project's success can be traced directly to a group of talented people who had a vision and saw it through.

So how does this tie back to fitness? Because when you're building a healthier and essentially ageless body, that foundation is muscle. There is no way I'd be able to handle the volume of my weekly workouts without a varied training routine—and a protein-centric diet—that produced strong muscles.

That's not to discount the heart, brain, lungs, or any other member of your cast of anatomical characters. Of course, you'll want all your organs, tissues, and systems functioning at top levels. But in terms of physical health—and of the benefits that come with it—a muscular base serves as the first block from which you build everything else. (And I would argue that having muscle helps all those other organs, tissues, and systems work better.) That's because muscle has so many benefits, especially as we age.

Remember: No matter how old or athletically challenged you are, you can change your body shape, your weight, your energy level, and other factors that will positively influence your quality of life by adding muscle to your body.

It's worth noting briefly how muscles work in relation to physical activity. When you perform a physical task—walking, lifting weights, chopping wood—muscle fibers are broken down, which is why you feel sore afterward. Your body then seeks to self-repair. When you're properly nourished, your body responds by building more muscle fibers in anticipation that you're going to try once again to stress your muscles. That process repeats itself the more you challenge your body. So when you regularly put your muscles under strain, they continue to fortify themselves. They gain in strength, which means they'll be up to the challenges even more so the next time.

There are countless reasons to build strength:

◆ Muscle supports your skeletal structure

Weight training can increase bone density. In the absence of exercise, bone density naturally diminishes as you age. Increased bone density can help prevent osteoporosis and reduce back pain, which affects four out of five Americans.

◆ Muscle is metabolically efficient

More energy is required to maintain muscle than to maintain fat, which means being more muscular can aid weight-loss efforts. In a study published in the *Scandinavian Journal of Clinical & Laboratory Investigation*, participants who performed one-hour training sessions three times a week for 12 weeks experienced an increase in resting metabolic rate (RMR), which decreases the risk of obesity and,

Good mornings start with good people.

—Zack Zeigler, 36, The Program

I met Zack when he and his wife, Erica Schultz (page 164), were covering The Program for a feature in *Muscle & Fitness* magazine—well before we began writing *Becoming Ageless* together. Their assignment was to arrive at Pier 46 in Manhattan at 6 a.m. to witness 30 of us take on one of Flex Cabral's notoriously brutal outdoor boot camps. Zack and Erica quickly found themselves hustling to keep up with and photograph the action. Zack's coworkers told him that we were a bunch of models who had created a "secret society" that required you to be shredded to join. Well, that wasn't true, but in The Program you do have to take your fitness seriously no matter what shape you're in.

After the workout, Zack interviewed members of the team and realized that the connection among the group, for both men and women, was deep and sincere. We asked Zack and Erica to join The Program—and it has changed Zack's approach to training. Keep in mind he's an editor at a fitness magazine.

"My workouts had become stale and unenjoyable. The Program introduced me to group training and prompted me to take inventory of my diet and daily routine," he says. "There's no denying that I'm in vastly better shape than when I started. But the group has also reminded me how important it is to be surrounded by positive, friendly, and motivated people. That's why on the days we train, 6 a.m. never comes too early—it doesn't come early enough."

according to the American Heart Association, helps prevent body-fat accumulation.

◆ Resistance training can increase your overall quality of life as you age

Researchers from Virginia Tech and Adelphi University found that resistance training can reduce insulin resistance and body fat, and improve RMR, glucose metabolism, and blood pressure—high levels of which are associated with diabetes, heart disease, and cancer. The benefits could be seen in as little as two 15- to 20-minute strength-training sessions per week (and without the use of superheavy weight). In addition, weight-bearing exercise has been shown to enhance mood and energy levels.

As is the case with nearly everything in the diet and fitness industry, there are multiple definitions of "strength training." As to which approach you should take—again, what do you want?

Assuming you're not training for the Olympics, NFL Combine, or a bodybuilding competition, you probably just want to sculpt a healthy, trim physique that looks good both in and out of clothing. One trap I would suggest you avoid is to compare yourself with cover models or people who are paid to remain fit. Instead, focus on continuous improvement.

Former NFL fullback Tony Richardson played in three Pro Bowls and was inducted into the Kansas City Chiefs Hall of Fame in 2016. Rob Pannell is a professional lacrosse player for the New York Lizards. Both incredibly athletic men are members of The Program. If I got frustrated every time Tony or Rob beat me in sprints, life wouldn't be enjoyable. When you compare yourself with others, in every instance, you will

APPROACH	WHAT TO KNOW
FREE WEIGHTS (BARBELLS, DUMBBELLS, KETTLEBELLS)	These are great options for a variety of traditional resistance exercises, including both full-body bilateral and unilateral movements. Using a spotter can help you avoid injury. You can add challenges to many exercises by changing up the mode (i.e., lifts you do with a barbell can be done with dumbbells to isolate each arm or leg separately).
WEIGHT MACHINES	Machines enforce strict form and remove the risk of dropping a weight on yourself. The downsides: You're less likely to engage your core muscles when using machines; not all body types are suited for machines; and proper adjustments can be difficult.
BODY-WEIGHT EXERCISES	Push-ups, pull-ups, air squats, mountain climbers, and lots of other options allow you to build muscle by moving your own body weight. These exercises can be incredibly challenging and engage your core. They also make up a good portion of the moves that I do in intensity-based workouts. Best of all, they require almost no equipment and can be done almost anywhere.
SUSPENSION TRAINERS	TRX and other suspension trainers allow you to pull, push, and hold your body in a variety of positions. These tools are long woven-fabric straps with handles on one end that are connected to a sturdy anchor point, such as a horizontal bar. They allow more options than traditional body-weight moves and engage your core in almost every exercise.
RESISTANCE BANDS	Bands provide tension and resistance as you push or pull them. These large elastic bands are great for traveling because you can stuff them in a carry-on, but unless you invest in thicker bands, they may not provide enough resistance as you progress. These are also good to use for stretching. Just be sure not to let go while the band is under tension; it's an easy way to get hurt.

find someone who is more competent than you at something—usually many things. That's why I try to maintain a healthy sense of humor about myself. It doesn't mean I won't try to outrun Rob, but I won't be super hard on myself if I gave it my all and still finished a second or two—OK, fine, three—after him, either.

Keeping that in mind, while you work to gain strength, research shows you'll also improve—and perhaps even lengthen—your life. Here's how to get started.

Start Slow

A TYPICAL SCENARIO for someone starting a new workout regimen looks like this: Get excited, hit the gym, lift heavy and for a long time, wake up the next day feeling horrible, and then avoid the gym for the foreseeable future. Remember, doing too much, too soon will send you back to the couch or the doctor's office rather than back to the gym. Increase your effort gradually. That applies to the weight you use, as well as to the time you spend in the gym. You can work up to a hard 45-minute session, but don't attempt it right away. If you're already active but want to step things up a bit, start with a 10-minute full-body circuit and slowly progress from there. If you're a true beginner or are returning from a very long hiatus, the Becoming Ageless Workout Plan (pages 210–221) is the perfect place to start.

Realize You Can Do More Than You Think

ONCE YOU'VE ESTABLISHED a foundation of strength after several months of resistance training, you might not need as much recovery time as some suggest. What I'm referring to is the oft-repeated notion that it always takes 48 hours for your muscles to recover after a strength-training session. Given how often I train, I'm basically working my muscles constantly. How do I do that and avoid injury? I eat well, prioritize sleep, and limit the toxins I put into my body. *That* is recovery.

I don't believe you should be lifting heavy five days a week or twice a day, every day, but you can do more than you think. And while the amount of volume in my weekly training schedule can be demanding—especially when I do two-a-days or the number of weekly workouts enters double digits—it's nowhere near that of a high-level athlete. Those men and women have incredibly taxing programs that include multiple training sessions through-out the week. With the right approach to nutrition and recovery, they're able to perform an incredible amount of volume, vastly more than any of us needs to be in great shape.

The first time I had a sense that I could do more than I thought had nothing to do with weight training, but it eventu-ally carried over. When I was a high-school student, I didn't apply myself. Unsurprisingly (to everyone except me), I didn't get into Harvard, the college I had my heart set on attending. It was the wake-up call I needed.

I chose to go to Wesleyan and saw results after applying effort to my studies. It was the first time in my life I excelled at something. I liked that feeling and have never lost the urge to excel since or forgotten that I'm capable of doing more than I think. In the end, your body is way tougher than your mind leads you to believe. Accept that you can do more, that you can withstand discomfort, and that your will might bend but will not break, and it will become your reality.

Push and Pull the Weight

BARBELLS, DUMBBELLS, AND kettlebells are all effective tools for measuring progress. After all, if you can lift more weight, you're getting stronger. But as long as you're pushing or pulling something—even your body weight—and subjecting your muscles to significant duress for a short period, you're building strength using resistance.

Use a Challenging Weight, Not an Absurd Weight

BUILDING MORE MUSCLE will boost strength and reduce body fat. The way to build more muscle is regularly to challenge your body to adapt. Ways to do this include changing variables such as equipment and intensity style, or by simply lifting more weight and adding more repetitions—what's known as adding "volume" to your workout. Use the same weight indefinitely and your body will adapt, leading to a plateau.

Determining the ideal set-and-rep approach can be tricky. Some experts advocate doing more sets using lighter weight for 15 to 20 reps, while others advise doing fewer sets and using heavier weight for three to five reps. Unless your training is highly sport-specific, the risk of going ultraheavy is most likely not worth the reward. That said, going superlight is probably not enough to optimize muscle growth. A study published in the *Journal of Strength and Conditioning Research* monitored two groups of lifters using either low- or high-load resistance training. After eight weeks, both groups increased muscle thickness. However, the group that did eight to 12 repetitions gained more strength than the group that did more reps using lighter weight.

You might have noticed how I didn't tell you that building muscle or strength hinges on your answer to the question: "How much do you bench?" That's not an interesting question or a true gauge of strength or power unless you're in a competition where the amount of weight you bench-press will benefit you. Otherwise, when you're trying to get fit and build an

> **"The way to change—and to sustain that change—is to take your time."**

aesthetically pleasing physique, there is no need to lift or press more and more weight. I've witnessed people spending an hour just on the bench press, lifting superheavy weight and contorting their bodies into positions that compromise form— it's a recipe for injury.

So what's the best approach to consistently build strength? Variety. If you're on a three-day resistance-training schedule, try the eight- to 12-rep approach for two days and a heavier five-set, five-rep approach for one day. Here's what to do:

Focus on Big Muscles

I ENJOY VARYING my workouts, but if my goal were solely to build strength and muscle, I'd focus on major muscle groups— chest, back, legs—to get the most metabolic impact. Training large muscle groups burns more energy. Big-muscle compound lifts like the squat, bench press, pull-up, and deadlift are the ones that really matter. A program consisting of only compound lifts, which involve more than one joint and muscle group, is enough to get you into great shape.

Do More Core Work

A STRONG CORE is about more than just having visible abs— nutrition and low body fat are much more responsible for that.

"Ultimately, intensity is pushing your mind's resistance to what your body can actually do."

A strong core provides the stability for high performance and a low injury rate, which is why it's a key component of any muscle-building program. While the rectus abdominis—the "six-pack muscle" running down your stomach—gets most of the attention, the core is actually made up of your abs (including the obliques), lower back, hips, and glutes.

I often finish my exercise routines with five to 10 minutes dedicated to core work. You should consider doing that, as well. It will pay dividends in every other area of fitness.

Use the Becoming Ageless Workout Plan

THE BEST AND safest approach for beginners or people living sedentary lives is simply to get moving—walk more, stretch, develop a greater range of motion, improve flexibility, and, most important, exercise patience. Remember that as long as you're getting more exercise than you were before, you're headed in the right direction.

Advance at a comfortable pace and aim to devote 12 weeks to the Becoming Ageless Workout Plan found on pages 210–221. It was designed to ease you gently into being active five to six days a week, with three of those days focused on full-body, weight-training workouts.

According to research published in the *Journal of Strength and Conditioning Research*, beginners are likely to see more desirable results regarding strength gains and body-fat reduction using this method than other training protocols, such as body-part-specific training. As your fitness level increases over time, you'll want to make it a habit to change things up every three to four weeks—use different equipment, fluctuate the volume, weight load, rest periods, etc. Doing so presents continuous challenges to the muscles and central nervous system; failing to do so will lead to stagnation.

For now, a basic routine that builds full-body strength is all you need. In the chart on the following page, your "Main Lifts" will primarily focus on the legs, back, and chest; the "Secondary Lifts" will aid strength gains in your Main Lifts while also working your shoulders, biceps, and triceps. The "Core Exercises" and "Body-Weight Exercises" are used to develop stability and balance, as well as work your abdominals.

THE *BECOMING AGELESS* EXERCISES

MAIN LIFTS (pages 222–227)	Bench Press, Incline Bench Press, Deadlift, Kettlebell Romanian Deadlift, Pull-Up, Lat Pulldown, Barbell Squat, Dumbbell Squat
SECONDARY LIFTS (pages 228–233)	Dumbbell Lunge, Dumbbell Overhead Press, Dumbbell Step-Up, Dumbbell Shrug, Dumbbell Lateral Raise, Triceps Rope Pushdown, Bentover Lateral Raise, Dumbbell Curl, Dumbbell Hammer Curl, Seated Overhead Triceps Extension
CORE EXERCISES (pages 234–235)	Push-Up, Bicycle, Plank, Leg Raise
BODY-WEIGHT MOVES (pages 236–237)	Russian Twist, Air Squat, Burpee

See exercise descriptions starting on page 222.

The Becoming Ageless Workout Plan kicks off with two weeks of body-weight moves, walking, and stretching. In Week 3 you'll perform your first strength circuit—one set, nine exercises, five to 10 reps for each. Regarding the weights you select, if you can't get five reps with perfect form, reduce the weight. If 10 reps are too easy, increase the weight.

By Week 12, you will have eased into doing three weekly training sessions that consist of three sets of 12 reps per exercise and three to five sets of five reps for a total of 45 minutes to one hour per session.

Perform a dynamic stretching routine for four to eight minutes to warm up your body before any strength workout.

CHAPTER 2

Find a Better Balance

Use dynamic stretches, foam rollers, and yoga to improve flexibility and increase strength.

DESPITE MY PASSION for fitness and the role it plays in my life, my wife isn't especially interested in it. In fact, Wendy has many times in the past—often but not always with a sense of humor—given me a hard time about how much I work out. But that hasn't stopped me from trying to include her. Usually, I'll suggest that we go to the gym, and she'll agree to "after taking care of a few things." So I'll wait. And wait some more. Eventually, she might say, "Maybe we should go get a coffee instead of going to the gym."

Together we came to an agreement that working out together wasn't the most uplifting experience for either of us. But I wasn't ready to give up. She'll deny this, but I firmly recall Wendy telling me that she liked yoga. So I signed us up for a yoga class, which turned out to be a hot power yoga class. We had no idea what we were getting into, but I went in with an open mind. As the temperature inside the room reached 105 degrees, everything clicked—the music, the atmosphere, the sweat, and the challenge meshed together to create an almost spiritual trance.

We walked out of the class, both dripping with sweat. We then looked at each other and spoke in unison:

"I'm never doing that again," she said.

"That was a religious experience," I said.

Suffice it to say, that was the last time Wendy sweated it out in a hot yoga class. (Still, as a deeply accomplished equestrienne and a devoted, indefatigable mother of three—and wife to a guy who routinely wakes her up at 5 a.m.—Wendy has proven to be plenty flexible without practicing hot yoga.)

While serious yoga practitioners generally look down on hot yoga—many view it as the watered-down McDonald's of yoga styles—I was drawn to it. Having done restorative, or slow, yoga a few times before, I wasn't impressed. Adding in the heat, the sweat, and the exercise element made for a gentle but challenging, low-intensity, highly rewarding hour that allowed me to find balance in my routines while serving as what felt like a spiritual unlocking. Now I can't imagine my weekly routine without a yoga session.

You'll find that a huge part of the Becoming Ageless Workout Plan is gaining a greater sense of balance. Not just the kind of balance that helps gymnasts excel—and not just yoga, either. Rather, balance in the form of your workout regimen:

combining high-intensity exercise, strength training, and gentle recovery and stretching routines. I now have a robust and diverse training approach that includes a good deal of preparation and recovery. This is reflected in my feeling more athletic and competent and stronger—not to mention that at age 60, my body probably looks better than it ever has. But finding the right balance took time.

Up until my 30s I didn't do any cardio work. I wasn't putting on weight, so why bother? The answer, as I would come to learn: Cardiovascular exercise is essential for heart health. And up until the past few years, I'd foam-roll or stretch pre- or post-workout only if it was part of a class or administered by a trainer. I was finally able to put all the pieces together and construct the coordinated approach you'll find starting on page 210, which will help your muscles recover, optimize your overall fitness, and reduce the risk of injury.

The *Becoming Ageless* Case for Balance

ALONG WITH INTENSITY and strength workouts, some combination of yoga, foam rolling, or dynamic stretching forms the third side of my fitness triangle. Dynamic stretching involves stretching while you move your body (as opposed to static stretches that keep you in a fixed position, such as touching your toes). You'll find the Becoming Ageless Stretching Routine on page 61.

There is some conflicting evidence as to whether stretching enhances performance or aids in injury prevention. Research out of the University of Hull in England reported that static stretching was ineffective for reducing exercise-related injuries, though there was some evidence to support that stretching reduced muscle-tendon injuries. Still, most athletic trainers advise a dynamic warm-up before exercising. That's what we do in The Program.

It's never too late to change the game.

—Tony Richardson, 46, The Program

Tony entered the NFL in the mid-1990s and spent 16 seasons playing fullback for the Kansas City Chiefs, Minnesota Vikings, and New York Jets before retiring in 2010. During that time Tony's weight training involved lots of heavy squats and bench presses. As part of his post-retirement fitness regimen, he was practicing at Pure Yoga, which is where we met. When Tony joined The Program, he was most compelled by the variety of workouts and the group dynamic—both of which helped him transform himself from a thick brick wall of a fullback to an overall fit guy.

"I don't miss the game, but I do miss the camaraderie," Tony says. "The Program workouts are great—game changers in a lot of areas of life. I've lost 15 to 20 pounds, and my body feels so much better. A 6 a.m. workout is better than the first cup of coffee."

I'd also suggest using a foam roller pre- and post-workout to relax away and iron out any knots or kinks from your muscles. A foam roller is a length of closed-cell foam about six inches in diameter and 18 to 36 inches in length. Basically, you place your weight on it, using any body part—from arms to glutes, thighs to upper back—and roll back and forth. Technically called myofascial release, what rolling provides is a self-massage that can be painful but is highly beneficial. A study published in the *Journal of Athletic Training* found that regular foam roller use reduced test subjects' muscle soreness, improved their range of motion, and increased their vertical-jump performance.

I've already told you how positive yoga has been for me both physically and spiritually, and science has found other ways in which practicing yoga can be beneficial:

Yoga Reduces Stress and Helps Manage Blood Pressure

A STUDY OUT of Arizona State University found that participants had significant improvements in blood pressure, muscular strength, perceived stress, and flexibility after just six weeks of yoga. Another study in the journal *Complementary Therapies in Medicine* reported that yoga could also help improve energy, happiness, social relationships, and sleep.

Exercise has been shown to reduce emotional exhaustion as well as boost self-confidence and mood for up to 12 hours post-workout. I'm basically always in a good mood, and I believe the amount, variety, and intensity of exercise in my weekly training regimen are big reasons for that.

Yoga Improves Flexibility and Balance

RESEARCHERS OUT OF Northeastern Illinois University and National University in San Diego discovered that athletes who practiced yoga performed better in various flexibility and balance tests than those who didn't.

Yoga Supports Gains in Strength

A 12-WEEK STUDY published in the *Journal of Strength and Conditioning Research* determined that when people developed a greater range of motion, it translated to greater muscle size and strength compared with subjects who used a partial range of motion during various squat exercises.

Yoga Combats Obesity

RESEARCH OUT OF the University of Arizona indicated that yoga could prevent obesity and diseases related to it. If you're not interested in yoga, stretching your muscles may offer many of the benefits you'd experience from a yoga session. Focus on moving through the full range of motion during each move.

THE BECOMING AGELESS
STRETCHING ROUTINE

Perform these flexibility stretches and yoga exercises in succession for 4 to 8 minutes on an off day, as part of a dynamic warm-up, or as your post-training cooldown.

NECK CIRCLE	Slowly roll your head in circles. Complete 10 reps in one direction and then repeat in the opposite direction.
SHOULDER CIRCLE	Stand with your feet shoulder-width apart, raise both arms overhead, and slowly make circles with your arms—10 reps clockwise, 10 reps counterclockwise. Do not rotate the wrists or elbows during the movement.
ANKLE CIRCLE	Lift one leg off the floor and rotate your ankle clockwise for 10 reps, then counterclockwise for 10 reps.
CHAIR POSE	Stand upright with your arms by your sides. Bend at the knees to get into a squat position, and raise your arms overhead while maintaining a flat back. Hold for 15 seconds. Do 5 reps.
HIGH LUNGE	Take a big step forward until the knee of your extended leg is just off the ground. Place your palms on the floor on both sides of your extended leg. Press the ball of your extended foot into the floor for a 10 count. Return to the start position and switch legs. Do 5 reps per leg.
DEEP SQUAT	Stand with feet hip-width apart, toes slightly pointed out. Keeping your chest up and torso upright, sink down into a squat as low as you comfortably can. Hold for 3 to 5 seconds, then return to the start position. Squeeze your glutes when you're standing upright.
GLUTE STRETCH	Lie flat on your back with your knees bent and your feet on the ground. Put your left ankle on your right knee. Now use your hands to pull your right knee toward your chest. Switch sides when you're done.
GLUTE BRIDGE	Lie on your back with both feet on the floor and your legs bent. Thrust your hips toward the ceiling as high as you can, squeezing your glutes. Return to the start position. Do 8 to 10 reps.

HOW I BALANCE MY WEEK

Because of travel and work obligations, my week-to-week workout schedule isn't always consistent. So while the training split listed below is typical of what my week looks like, things routinely shift around.

MONDAY

Morning: High-intensity weight training with a personal trainer (45 minutes)

Evening: Timed kettlebell workout with a friend (30 minutes)

TUESDAY

Morning: Hot power yoga with The Program (1 hour)

Evening: Rest or boxing class (1 hour)

WEDNESDAY

Morning: Running with The Program (1 hour)

Evening: High-intensity weight training with a personal trainer (45–60 minutes)

THURSDAY

Morning: High-intensity boot camp with The Program (45 minutes)

Evening: Stretching and body-weight work solo or with a friend (30–45 minutes)

FRIDAY

Morning/Evening: Circuit training with The Program (45 minutes)

SATURDAY

Morning/Evening: Rest or a slow-paced noncardio weight workout solo or with a friend (30–45 minutes)

SUNDAY

Morning/Evening: Rest or cycling (distances and times vary)

CHAPTER 3

Dial Up Your Intensity

Know the science behind high-intensity workouts, how to ease into them, and how best to build your own explosive routine.

I AM MY HARSHEST CRITIC—personally, professionally, athletically—but when I fall short knowing I gave maximum effort, I don't dwell on it. So, when I made it a goal over the past several years to train with people who are half my age, I accepted that I might not finish first, execute the most reps, or lift the most weight, but I insisted on working as hard as possible. And while The Program isn't filled with Olympians, each person takes fitness seriously, and that fuels the entire collective to work harder to achieve results.

In the past, I believed that people who were in good shape were genetically superior and that maintaining their lean or healthy status required little to no effort. But after training with a motivated group whose members aim to improve and exert as much effort during their workouts as I do, I've found that even though I'm not genetically gifted, I'm still able to get into good shape and train at a high level.

Hands down, the most physically demanding workout The Program does is on Thursday mornings at Trooper Fitness, a studio gym in the Midtown East section of Manhattan. It's not a big space—maybe the size of a large living room—and there's not a lot of equipment, either. Some bars, mats, hurdles, ropes, kettlebells, and a few other fitness toys. About 15 to 20 of us can cram into the room for a 45-minute session with Flex Cabral, a former Marine who ushers us through a sweat-inducing, nonstop shoulders-to-calves workout. The routines vary from week to week but usually involve a combination of pushing, pulling, jumping, and aerobics. Sometimes we use weights, other times it's body weight only. Regardless, once we start, we go. Each exercise is followed by another, with just enough rest to transition—starting with an intense, physically demanding warm-up.

Flex routinely changes the protocol and exercises to ensure that each session is just as tough or tougher than the previous one—and that's what makes his classes so enjoyable. This style of training embodies everything that is right with exercise: It's intense, efficient, and effective.

But what *is* intensity, anyway? And how do you measure it?

Let's start with what intensity isn't. Many beginners equate an *intense* workout with their level of corresponding soreness afterward. That's not your best or most accurate measure of determining whether a workout was a success. For example, years ago I ran a 5K race without training for it or even running for a year. But since I had been cycling three days per week and my recovery efforts were adequate, I felt I'd be fine. The good news: I finished the race. The bad news: My extreme soreness prevented me from training for the next week.

Had I eased my way into the training—even jogging a couple of miles on a consistent basis—I would not have experienced such horrible soreness. But a little stiffness—also known as delayed onset muscle soreness (DOMS), a common but uncomfortable feeling people experience while the body repairs itself—isn't necessarily bad. It serves as a reminder that muscle tissue has been damaged and that I need to eat and rest properly before my next training session, which, if the DOMS is too intense, may involve a full day of rest.

If you're a true beginner, don't push yourself too hard, too quickly. When you reach a point where you consider yourself fit and have the ability or urge to expand outside of your comfort zone, go for it. But not on Day 1.

Your progress with "steady-state activities"—exercise performed at a constant speed for a set period, such as mild jogging or rowing—is reflected in distance or speed. With weight training, you see progression in loads. Intensity, in many ways, is measured by *feel*—that is, the burn in your quads and biceps on your twenty-fifth burpee or when your tired mind and body consider walking the last few steps of a six-story stair run. Ultimately, intensity is pushing your mind's resistance to what your body can actually do.

"A muscular base serves as the first block from which you build everything else."

Once you're comfortable doing that, you can aim to progress incrementally and continuously. How will you know you're progressing? If you feel better after your last set of push-ups or stair runs today than you did the previous week, you're improving. These types of mini-markers can provide a real sense of accomplishment and drive you to do more.

Don't be hard on yourself if you don't advance immediately. Try to remember that you chose this activity because you enjoy it. Even if you're not as adroit as you'd like to be, you can and will work up to being competent if you don't give up. I speak from experience.

About eight years ago I decided to add a new component to my fitness routine that would take me out of my comfort zone—boxing. I went to a trainer at Mendez Boxing in New York City, a no-frills gym straight out of *Rocky*—beat-up heavy bags hanging from the ceiling, title-fight promo posters and photos of iconic fighters such as Ali, Tyson, and Pacquiao hanging in frames on the wall. It was gritty, smelly, and filled with skilled fighters and coaches. My first task wasn't to throw a punch—it was to jump rope repeatedly. Even after a few weeks, my performance was hardly Ali-worthy—I tripped repeatedly. One of the old trainers watched, smiled, and said, "First time, eh?" In the end, it took me three months to jump rope reasonably well.

Mentally overcoming that obstacle was a challenge, but the physical component was equally daunting. Most of the workouts involve three minutes of nonstop heavy bag, speed bag, or pad work, followed by one minute of active rest. Active rest isn't the same as "rest," either. You're doing things like burpees, push-ups, or squat jumps to keep your heart rate elevated. Acquiring the coordination and skill to complete the drills and build up the stamina to make it through the grueling boxing workout was something I had to get used to. But I stayed with it because, as hard as you work during the session, you feel that much better when you're done. That's something people often forget.

It may seem counterintuitive, but the wiped-out feeling I experience directly after a boxing or high-intensity workout improves my energy, enables me to manage stress, and enhances my leadership at the office. My friend Jay Hass (page 39) said it perfectly: "When I get through a hard workout, everything else is easy."

There is plenty of evidence to show improved health and general fitness with steady-state cardio exercise such as jogging on a treadmill. I used to do plenty of it, especially cycling, and now and then I still do—mostly for relaxation and recovery. But, as science demonstrates, there are plenty of reasons why you should engage in intense physical activity as you move closer to *Becoming Ageless.*

Here are the best ways to do it:

Build an Intensity-based Workout

WHEN FOLLOWING A HIIT protocol—for example, 20 seconds of sprinting followed by 10 seconds of walking—you'll spend your working sets pushing yourself and the recovery time taking it easy. This pacing allows you to give maximum effort and also recharge before the next challenge.

What makes HIIT (see pages 40–42 for some background) even more appealing is that it's time-efficient, which is ideal for busy people. Sometimes work or family obligations determine how long I have to train, and a quick-hitting, full-body HIIT session gets the job done. Research backs this up: A six-week study published in the journal *PLOS ONE* had sedentary, overweight or obese men train with HIIT or moderately intense exercise. At the end of the study, the HIIT subjects were found to have lower body-fat percentages, making it a more time-efficient training approach, despite having spent 20 percent less time working out.

I use a variety of intensity methods when I exercise, but I encourage beginners to start slow and experiment with sets, reps, rest, and work time that complement their fitness and comfort levels. Begin with 10 minutes of a steady-state cardiovascular activity like walking, running, swimming, rowing, elliptical training, or biking twice a week. Build to three times per week and add time as you improve. Once you hit the

5 REASONS TO RAMP UP THE INTENSITY

1) **You'll lose weight.**
   A study published in the journal *Metabolism* found that subjects who engaged in steady-state endurance training expelled twice as much energy but didn't lose as much weight as the subjects who trained with high intensity.

2) **You'll lose abdominal fat.**
   Researchers from the U.S. and France found that an eight-week intensity program among middle-aged men with type 2 diabetes resulted in a 44 percent reduction in abdominal fat compared with the control group. (They also increased thigh muscle by 24 percent.)

3) **Your cardiovascular health will improve.**
   In a study published in *PLOS ONE*, women with a syndrome associated with insulin resistance were randomly assigned to one of three groups—high-intensity interval training (HIIT), strength training, or a control group. After 10 weeks, both exercise groups experienced significant body-fat decreases, but only the women who did HIIT three times a week improved their blood sugar control, raised HDL (good) cholesterol levels, and increased the flexibility of their veins, improving blood flow—all markers of better cardiovascular health.

4) **Your strength will increase.**
   Researchers from the University of Jyvaskyla in Finland compared the strength of men who habitually sprinted with nonathletic men and found that the sprinters had 21 percent greater strength.

5) **Your overall performance will improve.**
   A study published in the *Journal of Sports Medicine & Physical Fitness* looked at the effects of uphill sprint training on soccer players. A sprinting group improved in speed drills, strength, and agility, while the performance of a nonsprinting group remained the same.

30-minute mark, it's time to add high-intensity periods into your cardio routine.

See pages 81–83 for a list of HIIT routines.

Get in More Intense Cardio Sessions

SPRINTING IS ONE of the best ways to boost your metabolism. A study conducted by researchers from the University of Glasgow found that four to six 30-second sprints for six sessions resulted in significant decreases in waist and hip circumferences compared with the baseline. You can apply this research to all forms of exercise.

Despite having a runner's build growing up, I dreaded running because I wasn't very good at it. On a scale of 1 to 10, running for me was a minus 4. So in 2016, I took action. I hired a coach to teach me proper form and to force me to run. Originally he suggested regular one-hour sessions. I said I wanted to start with 45 minutes once a week, because I didn't want to hate it so much that I would stop. The first sessions consisted of sprints, longer-paced runs, and intervals. Physically, they were absolutely brutal. We started in November and continued throughout the winter. It took a few months, but seeing improvements added enjoyment and pushed those weekly workouts to a 6 on the scale. And my efforts were rewarded with a compliment from one of my friends and workout partners, Nick Sizer (page 157), who told me, "You no longer look like you've actually been shot when you run now."

Thanks, Nick.

What follows are some ideas for ways to structure high-intensity aerobic activities after your preferred method of warming up. Remember to cool down or stretch afterward. Wear a stopwatch to time yourself. Keep in mind that even if you have only 10 to 15 minutes, any cardio session for any duration of time is better than skipping a workout altogether.

FAST AND FURIOUS

Alternate between short bursts of maximum effort and active rest, where you perform a low or moderate version of the same activity.

RUN

Sprint as fast as you can for 30 seconds, then jog slowly for 45 seconds.

Do 6 times.

CYCLE

Cycle as fast as you can for 1 minute, then do a light spin for 90 seconds.

Do 10 times.

SWIM

Swim as fast as you can for 50 meters, then rest for 30 seconds.

Do 10 times.

PYRAMID

Pick an intensity level or pace that you can sustain for the longest work set. Try to maintain that for all your work sets.

RUN

- Run ¼ mile, then do a light jog for 2 minutes.
- Run ½ mile, then do a light jog for 2 minutes.
- Run ¾ mile, then do a light jog for 2 minutes.
- Run ½ mile, then do a light jog for 2 minutes.
- Run ¼ mile, then do a light jog for 2 minutes.

CYCLE

- Cycle ½ mile, then do a light spin for 2 minutes.
- Cycle 2 miles, then do a light spin for 2 minutes.
- Cycle 1 mile, then do a light spin for 2 minutes.
- Cycle ½ mile, then do a light spin for 2 minutes.

SWIM

- Swim 100 meters, then rest for 1 to 2 minutes.
- Swim 200 meters, then rest for 1 to 2 minutes.
- Swim 400 meters, then rest for 1 to 2 minutes.
- Swim 200 meters, then rest for 1 to 2 minutes.
- Swim 100 meters, then rest for 1 to 2 minutes.

ADVANCED

These workouts will help you find the zone between short bursts of all-out effort and a long, easy pace. You'll be forced to find a slightly uncomfortable pace and then maintain it. Try to maintain the same pace or speed for all your work sets.

RUN

Run hard for 400 meters, then jog for 400 meters.
Do 6 times.

CYCLE

Cycle hard for 2 miles, then do a light spin for 2 minutes.
Do 6 times.

SWIM

Swim hard for 200 meters, then use a slower pace for 50 meters.
Do 6 times.

ADD INTENSITY TO BODY-WEIGHT EXERCISES

Strength and intensity are entwined—meaning that you can (and should) do intense workouts that involve strength moves. I often pair body-weight moves—air squats, push-ups, pull-ups, and burpees (see exercise descriptions on pages 236, 234, 225, and 237)—together to form full-body circuit training, which is especially effective when you execute them using intervals.

Here's how to add intensity to these exercises and any body-weight strength workout. Mix and match and work in as many methods as you like for as little as 10 minutes or as much as an hour.

TABATA

Tabata training uses a 2-to-1 work-to-rest ratio. It's fun and energetic, and it works. Timed workouts are also phenomenal because they remove the risk of lack of compliance. You have to comply with the timer and don't have the option to think about, "When am I starting? When am I stopping? What am I doing?"

DO IT
Perform an exercise as hard and fast as you can for 20 seconds, then rest for 10 seconds. Repeat that format—20 seconds on, 10 seconds off—8 times for a total of 4 minutes. Then rest for 1 minute before the next exercise. Complete all four body-weight exercises listed above in this manner, omitting pull-ups if you're at home and don't have access to a pull-up bar.

ADD INTENSITY TO BODY-WEIGHT EXERCISES

100s

Doing 100s—in which you complete 100 reps of an exercise—isn't easy but makes for a great workout finisher.

DO IT
Perform 100 reps of each exercise. Use a rest-pause method, in which you do as many reps as possible, rest for 10 to 15 seconds, and then continue until you reach the 100-rep mark. Or mix and match—20 squats, 25 push-ups, 10 burpees, and so on—until you complete 100 reps of each move.

If 100 reps isn't challenging enough, step it up with Barbara, one of the few CrossFit Workouts of the Day that I enjoy: Perform 5 rounds for time, resting 3 minutes between rounds:

20 pull-ups
30 push-ups
40 sit-ups
50 squats

ADD INTENSITY TO
BODY-WEIGHT EXERCISES

EMOM

"Every Minute on the Minute" (EMOM) is a great method to use when you're crunched for time. The rest periods help keep you accountable; the longer it takes to get through your set, the less rest you have. You'll be active and changing things up every minute to keep things lively.

DO IT
Pick a number of reps for each exercise (say, 15 push-ups, 20 squats, etc.). Do 15 push-ups, then rest until the minute is up. When the next minute starts, do 20 squats, then rest. Start with 10 minutes. Keep cycling through the exercises for 20 minutes.

PLAYING CARDS

When my training feels repetitive, this never fails to reignite my motivation. Don't be fooled by the simplicity: The volume creeps up on you and the randomness of the cards tricks your mind into compliance.

DO IT
Match one exercise for each card suit. (Heart is for burpees, spade is for push-ups, etc.) Select a card and perform that number of reps for that designated exercise. With a partner, alternate picks until you run out of cards. Aces equal 11 reps; face cards are 15; a joker is a 400-meter run.

BOXING MOVES

No sparring necessary. Hitting a heavy bag or speed bag or repping out punches or combos will make you pour sweat. However, I'd recommend taking a private lesson or two at a boxing gym to learn punching mechanics. If you don't have a heavy bag or speed bag, then shadowbox. Here are some basics that will help you get started:

Stance: Stand with your feet about shoulder-width apart and staggered (back heel aligned with your front toes). Bend your knees slightly and angle your body to one side and turn your front foot out 45 degrees, back foot out 30 degrees. Keep your weight evenly distributed and your upper body relaxed and loose with your hands at eye level, chin tucked to shoulder, and elbows tight to the body.

Jab: With your nondominant hand (this shoulder should be closest to the bag), snap your arm out as far as you can, taking a little step with your lead foot. Keep your dominant hand at face level (to protect your face, theoretically).

Cross: After throwing two or three jabs, uncoil your hip and punch the bag with your dominant hand, driving it from behind you through the bag. This is the power punch.

Hook: Aim to make contact with the side of the bag with your arm moving parallel to the floor and your elbow bent about 90 degrees. Initiate the movement with your hips in the direction you're punching, pivot your feet toward the target, and keep your wrist in line with your elbow as you make contact with the bag.

Uppercut: Shift your weight to your front foot, dip your front shoulder, pivot on the balls of your feet, and explode upward as you deliver the punch. Try not to drop your rear hand.

BOXING MOVES

HEAVY-WEIGHT BOUT
Shadowbox or punch a heavy bag for 3 minutes, then rest for 1 minute.

Do 3 times.

TABATA
Rapid-fire, hard punches for 20 seconds, 10 seconds of rest for 4 minutes.

Do 2 times.

TRAINING SESSION
Punch for 3 minutes, rest for 1 minute, jump rope for 3 minutes, rest for 1 minute.

Do 2 times.

ADVANCED
Buy boxing gloves and pads so you're punching to a partner's hands, not just the bag. You can do combos—jab, cross, hook, uppercut—and even integrate squats as you duck your partner's faux punches.

Structure the workout based on time or follow a Tabata protocol.

Do 4 times.

COMBINATIONS

Exercise should always be challenging and surprising—never boring. Mix and match all the elements previously discussed. Use time, style, and reps as variables and you can create infinite ways to structure an efficient, effective, and intense workout.

Here are some examples:

COMBO 1
- 3 minutes of punching
- 20 air squats
- 10 burpees
- 15 push-ups
- ¼-mile run (treadmill, stairs, or outdoors)
- Rest for 1 minute
- Do 3 times

COMBO 2
- Tabata of burpees (20 seconds on, 10 seconds off) for 8 rounds
- 2 minutes of cycling on a spinning bike (high resistance, simulating a hill)
- Rest for 1 minute
- Tabata of push-ups (20 seconds on, 10 seconds off) for 8 rounds
- 3 minutes of jumping rope
- Rest for 1 minute
- Do 2 times

COMBO 3
- 10 push-ups
- 10 burpees
- 25 air squats
- 1-minute treadmill run or erg (rowing machine)
- Rest for 1 minute
- Do 6 times

A little bit of support goes a long way.

—Dyan Tsiumis, 40, The Program

Dyan grew up during the fat-free craze and adopted a diet consisting largely of baked potatoes and fat-free honey mustard. She was an athlete in her youth, but describes her body then as "thick." Her passion for fitness led her to a major in athletic training in college. When she graduated, she stopped playing sports (and started partying). Dyan soon weighed nearly 200 pounds.

Having decided to make a change, she began to work out twice a day. At the same time, she became fascinated by the connection between mind and body, as well as the power of positive affirmation. She became a certified trainer, fitness instructor, and holistic health coach and was introduced to The Program when the team came to her indoor cycling class. Soon, Dyan was hooked on both the exercise and the camaraderie.

"It's not a competitive environment. It's super supportive," she says. "A few years ago, I did a bikini competition, and about 30 people from The Program showed up. Everyone looks out for one another and has each other's back."

DYNAMIC WARM-UP

The Program's workouts at Trooper Fitness are humbling and keep me and the team on our toes every week. Flex Cabral begins class with a dynamic stretch, which is defined as stretching and warming up your body through movement. Along with a dynamic stretch routine, I've included three of Flex's HIIT circuits.

Directions: Perform each move for 30 seconds unless otherwise noted.

SHIN TAP	Stand tall with feet shoulder-width apart. With left toes pointed up, lift up left leg and tap shin or knee with opposite hand. After 15 seconds, repeat with the right leg.
CRAWL OUT	Stand tall, bend over to place your hands on the floor, and "walk" your hands out to the plank position, then crawl back with your hands to the starting position.
UPWARD DOG	Lie on your stomach so your thighs and the tops of your feet are touching the floor. Place both hands palms-down on the floor at about chest level. Push your upper body up so that your back arches.
DOWNWARD DOG	Place your hands and feet on the floor so your body forms an inverted V. Aim to keep your knees as straight as possible (but don't lock them out). If you're not flexible enough for this pose, start by touching your toes, then progress to placing your palms on the floor.
WORLD'S GREATEST STRETCH	Get into a deep lunge position and place the hand opposite of your extended leg on the floor. Do not allow your rear knee to touch the floor as you rotate your torso toward your extended leg and drive the elbow back as deep as possible. Hold, then slowly return to the start position; repeat for 40 seconds. Then switch sides.

DYNAMIC WARM-UP

MOUNTAIN CLIMBER

Get into a push-up position with your arms straight. Your body should form a straight line from head to heels. Lift your right foot off the floor and bring your knees as close to your chest as you can. Touch the floor with your right foot and then return to the start position. Do the same with your left leg and continue alternating legs for 45 seconds.

SQUAT THRUST

Standing tall, bend down and put your hands on the floor in front of you, donkey-kick your feet behind you, and then hop your feet to your hands so that you are in a squat position. Stand up and repeat.

HIGH KNEES

Run in place, raising your knees toward your chest.

HIIT CIRCUIT I

Perform 1 set of each exercise and then move on to the next exercise. Rest for 10 to 15 seconds between exercises. Do 3 rounds.

ALTER-NATING JUMP LUNGE

Get into a lunge position with your left leg forward, thigh parallel with the floor, and your right leg behind you, knee bent at a right angle and hovering about an inch above the floor. Jump vertically and switch legs, landing softly while executing a lunge with your right leg forward; continue alternating sides.

Do the exercise for 45 seconds.

RUN

Run down (or up) 6 flights of stairs, run around the block outside, and then run back up (or down) 6 flights of stairs.

Or run on a treadmill at a moderate to high pace for 4 minutes.

PUSH-UP

Place your hands on the floor roughly shoulder-width apart. Your arms should be straight and your back should form a straight line from head to heels. Bend your arms to lower your body nearly to the floor while keeping your elbows close to your body. Aim to keep your body in a straight line throughout the movement. Don't allow your hips to sag.

Do the exercise for 45 seconds.

SQUAT JUMP

Stand with your feet slightly wider than shoulder width. Keep your chest up as you squat down until your thighs are parallel with the floor, then explode up and jump as high as you can. Land softly and lower yourself back into the squat position.

Do the exercise for 30 seconds.

HIIT CIRCUIT II

Perform 1 set of each exercise and then move on to the next exercise—except burpees, for which you will follow a Tabata format—20 seconds on, 10 seconds off, for 8 rounds. Rest 10 to 15 seconds between exercises. Do 1 to 3 rounds.

QUICK FEET

Starting with knees slightly bent, run in place rapidly, lifting feet just slightly off the floor, for 20 seconds.

RUN

Run down (or up) 6 flights of stairs, run around the block outside, and then run back up (or down) 6 flights of stairs.

Or run on a treadmill at a moderate to high pace for 4 minutes.

TUCK JUMP

Jump as high as you can and bring your knees to your chest at the top of the jump. Land softly, then jump again. Continue for 45 seconds.

BURPEE (TABATA)

Squat down and plant your hands on the floor, then donkey-kick your legs directly back into a push-up position, and then do a push-up. Hop your feet back to your hands, then explosively jump as high as you can, swinging your arms up toward the ceiling. Land softly.

HIIT CIRCUIT III

Perform 1 set of each exercise and then move on to the next exercise.
Rest 10 to 15 seconds between exercises. Do 3 rounds.

PULL-UP
Hang from a bar with your hands just outside shoulder width and your palms facing forward. Squeeze your shoulder blades together as you pull yourself up. Aim to get your chin over the bar. If the move proves too difficult, do assisted pull-ups or lat pulldowns.

Do 10 reps.

PUSH-UP
Place your hands on the floor at shoulder width. Brace your core and lower your body until your chest is about an inch above the floor. Press yourself back to the start position.

Do 10 reps.

CANDLE-STICK
Lie on the floor on your back and raise your legs toward the ceiling. Lift your glutes off the floor and extend your legs high.

Do 10 reps.

RUN
Run around the block.

Or run on a treadmill at a moderate to high pace for 4 minutes.

Age is just a number.

—Paul Schnell, 55, The Program

"Paul, you've put on eight pounds this year," the doctor said. It was the wake-up call Paul needed. He began training four days a week, and the weight vanished.

Paul works out with The Program three days a week. He also spins, plays basketball, and, depending on the time of year, plays tennis or skis.

"The whole has to be bigger than the parts. You want to build a culture where everyone is rooting for each other in the same direction," he says. "Being old is a mind-set. My dad skied until he was 83, and into his late 80s he also played golf and tennis, danced at parties, worked a few days per week, and lived every day with a bounce in his step—despite a persistent battle with cancer. Fitness has always been a journey with no destination. It's a way of life that combines the goal of mirroring my dad's joie de vivre, the desire to act and feel appropriately youthful, and to achieve a sense of accomplishment."

A BEGINNER'S GUIDE TO STRENGTH

STEP 1:   Remember that building strength, adding muscle, or getting lean overnight is not realistic. Be gentle on yourself and begin by making small changes that are low effort, high impact: Walk more, stretch more, and find ways to incorporate exercise into your weekly routine. Refer to the Becoming Ageless Workout Plan starting on page 210 for a detailed approach that starts slow and allows you to progress at your own pace.

STEP 2:   In the gym, select weights that are manageable but challenging and employ a variety of training styles. Focus primarily on compound exercises as your main lifts to strengthen your major muscle groups—back, chest, and legs—but do not neglect your core. If you can find a group of supportive and motivated people to train with, that's even better.

STEP 3:   Add intensity to your workout sessions by increasing the number of sets and reps, cutting rest periods, and using HIIT, Tabata, or any other method found on pages 70–83. Placing new demands on your muscles will help you avoid monotony and stagnation.

WHAT'S NEXT: Gradually build up to three intense weight-training sessions per week and make a point to incorporate other forms of exercise, including yoga, cycling, swimming, etc., into your schedule. Following the Becoming Ageless Workout Plan will get you there in about 12 weeks.

Part Two

EAT FOREVER FUEL

The best foods for getting lean,
fit, and muscular

86

SHORTLY AFTER BECOMING president and CEO at 20th Century Fox in 1989, I had a breakfast meeting, and I wanted to make a good impression. Only I didn't, and it wasn't because of a poorly chosen tie or a flimsy handshake. It was my order: two eggs over easy, white toast, bacon on the side, and a tall glass of orange juice. The guy I was meeting with ordered egg whites, blueberries, and black coffee, and he flashed a look of utter disgust at what I was putting into my body. Looking back, I should have shown restraint and *at least* gone with the small OJ. But in my 30s my diet was never something I scrutinized. In fact, up until my mid-50s it wouldn't be out of the question for me to eat pancakes for breakfast, pasta and a pastry for lunch, and something breaded for dinner with a slice of chocolate cake for dessert. Regardless of my exercise regimen, I've always needed to eat massive quantities of food to avoid weight loss. Formally, I'm what's referred to as an ecto-morph; colloquially, it'd be "hardgainer." Both terms mean the same thing: Adding muscle or gaining weight presents a chal-lenge. Even so, I was told my metabolism would slow down when I reached 30. It didn't. Forty? Nope. At 50, I noticed a change, but all that meant was that I had to scale back on quan-tities to avoid modest weight gain.

I knew the saying, "Abs are made in the kitchen," but that *still* wasn't enough. Only after I had reassessed my goals and decided that my midsection was to become a priority did I make changes—and that happened only after a trainer told me something I already knew: A toned midsection is all about diet. That's when it clicked, and I realized that I had been rejecting the notion despite knowing how obviously true it was. So it's from experience that I tell you that no exercise program can offset a diet heavy in doughnuts, pasta, and sugary fruit juice.

Along with weight gain, the damage you can inflict on your body with unhealthy food is vastly more profound than any gains you can achieve through exercise. That's simple caloric math. Unless your day job is working out, your body can't burn energy at the rate that you can consume it.

I think the diet industry has failed us when it comes to selling diet programs and products by telling us that you can eat what you want and still stay slim and fit. It's false. Here's the cold, hard truth: The food part can be difficult, and you'll need to make sacrifices. Heaping bowls of ice cream do not line the pathway to a lean, strong body.

If you want all the good things that come with being healthy and energetic, then you'll have to make better food choices. It's why, even though I'm eating clean to complement my intense fitness regimen, I regularly remind myself of my goals some 29 years after that business breakfast in L.A.

"The problem is that liquid calories all go down so fast, you hardly notice them."

The way I've structured the Becoming Ageless diet principles (pages 92–95) should allow you to categorize healthy and unhealthy foods easily while providing you with plenty of options for customization. But, again, it all comes down to your fitness goals. If you want to look like a fitness model—and your genetics support it—then you'll need to manage your diet tightly and train hard at least six days a week. But if you just want to get into really good shape, lose weight, and look lean, working out three or four days a week and eating a balanced diet and managing your calories will get the job done. And the easiest way to manage your calories is to manage your portions.

In the Becoming Ageless Eating Plan (pages 176–180), I will outline a plan for eating and drinking that—in conjunction with a solid training routine—will help you get the body you want. That plan is essentially based on the simple principle that if you burn more calories than you consume, you won't get fat. And if you consume more than you burn, you will. But there's more to the story. Nutrition expert Dr. Attia explains it well: "It's not just the calories; it's the chemistry. Different macronutrients— protein, carbohydrates, fat—trigger hormones differently. Some of those hormones promote fat storage, and some do not."

The trouble, at least for marketers who want to sell "one size fits all" programs, is there is no "one size fits all" reaction to macronutrient consumption. After working closely with Dr. Attia to determine what works best for me, I created an eating plan that provides a foundation for developing a healthy and strong life that should work for most people. You may need to adjust it as you see and feel how your body responds, but the main point is to consume the macronutrients that work in your favor and avoid the ones that don't. I do pay attention to calories in that I avoid empty calories or highly caloric foods when I can find a healthier substitute. For example, I'll exchange oily or creamy salad dressings in favor of a little lemon juice and vinegar.

Initially, minor dietary changes like that don't appear to accomplish much. Until you look at each one as a piece in a bigger puzzle: A large collection of small changes will support weight management and muscle building, as well as help keep your blood pressure in check and lower your risk of developing chronic diseases, such as cancer, heart disease, and diabetes.

Strive for consistency, not shortcuts.

—Mark Gerson, 45, The Program

In late 2001, Mark and his friend Cory Booker, who at the time was just starting his first run for mayor of Newark, New Jersey, agreed to a friendly bet over who could lose more weight. Mark took the wager seriously, slashing his caloric intake from 6,500 to 8,000 calories a day to 2,500 per day. Unsurprisingly, the weight came off quickly. Today, Mark weighs 165 pounds and runs almost every day. His diet centers on chicken, turkey, egg whites, hot sauce, and (occasionally) low-calorie ice cream and frozen yogurt. He doesn't consume red meat, most breads, potatoes, anything fried, or any liquids that contain calories.

"The fundamental rule of the diet is consistency," Mark says. "I apply to it what Stephen King wrote about writing. He used to tell interviewers that he wrote every day except for his birthday, the Fourth of July, and Christmas. Later he admitted that was a lie to make the interviews interesting and not sound 'like a workaholic dweeb.' The truth is that he does write every day. This consistency is as important for a formerly overweight person (at least this formerly overweight person) dealing with weight maintenance as it is for Stephen King. The body doesn't know if it's your birthday, Fourth of July, or Christmas any more than Stephen King's manuscripts do. So I consume the same number of calories (within, probably, a 10% band) every day."

CHAPTER 4

Your New Power Plate

Here's how, when, and what to eat
to ensure that you're loading up
on all the perfect foods for
building muscle and feeling great.

IDON'T BELIEVE I can ask much more of myself in terms of my commitment to fitness. My diet, however, continues to be a work in progress.

I feel as though it's important to reveal that this is true because I don't want to pretend that I embody perfection in any area of life, especially my dietary habits. I am friends with fitness models and fit people who proclaim they eat healthy 100 percent of the time, or that "it's easy" to adopt a mind-set in which raw salad and vegetables seem just as tasty as cakes and cookies. I'm skeptical of those claims because I also know fitness models and fit people who say those things in interviews but then eat sweets on a nightly basis. Besides, when you're paid to work out and you put in five to six hours per day at the gym, you can afford an extra cookie or two.

While I know there is room for improvement, what helps keep me steady is to remind myself of Dr. Attia's favorite analogy, which is to think of the body as a car and food as what fuels it. If you're looking to get from here to there, and how well or how long your car performs is of no concern, what you put into it won't matter much. For those of us who prefer to own a high-performance vehicle, the right fuel, the right maintenance, and the right team of mechanics are top priorities.

The thing is, as Dr. Attia explains, the exact type and amount of fuel needed varies from person to person. While some fundamental principles can guide your nutrition choices—a diet void of protein and high in saturated fat and sugar will leave you feeling sluggish and without your ideal body—finding the right ratios for each macronutrient will require experimentation. Since protein is key "forever fuel" for an ageless body, we'll take a closer look at 25 high-quality choices later in this chapter (pages 101–110).

The *Becoming Ageless* Diet Principles

I'VE ATTEMPTED TO make these tenets as simple as possible by breaking the nutrition guidelines into three categories— unlimited, limited, and highly restricted. This premise serves as the foundation for any healthy eating plan: Eat a lot of the foods that are clearly good for you and low in calories; eat some of the foods that are good for you but are higher-calorie; eat none or very few of the foods that are bad for you. Same goes for drinks. Apply the same guidelines and premise to your beverage choices each day.

DRINKS

UNLIMITED	Water, coffee, tea, seltzer (no added sodium).
LIMITED	Alcohol. (Sorry, red wine is actually not good for you. Alcohol is a toxin.)
HIGHLY RESTRICTED	Regular and diet soda; fruit and vegetable juice.

Aim to Eat Only Three Meals a Day

ADOPTING AND THEN sticking with a three-meals-a-day plan is going to be a challenge—especially for those of you who enjoy snacking. My food journal showed me just how detrimental my snacking habit had become. Eliminating foods that contain refined carbohydrates was particularly helpful. Those types of carbs digest quickly, can spike insulin, and initiate an up-and-down sensation of hunger, mood, and energy.

First, I relegated sweets and other snack foods made with refined carbs to cheat days. Then I eliminated unplanned snacking and built an optional snack into my daily food plan, which included things like 20 almonds, apple slices with PB2 powdered peanut butter, and a protein smoothie. (See my recipes starting on page 182.) Trust me, it wasn't—and still isn't—easy. And the temptation to snack doubles when I'm tired or traveling. But as tough as it's been, I have found that eating three meals a day—each made up of a moderate but filling amount of protein and limited amounts of healthy fats (avocado and nuts) and carbs (sweet potato and brown rice)—keeps me adequately fueled and feeling satiated.

Some diets advocate eating six small meals per day to help manage hunger and to keep your metabolism operating contin-

UNLIMITED

Protein: Especially lean protein, such as eggs, chicken breast, fish, lean red meat. Cap your intake at or around 1 gram per pound of body weight if you're trying to put on muscle. You can determine your recommended dietary allowance (RDA) for protein by multiplying your body weight in pounds by 0.36.

Salad: Use regular dressing sparingly. Try lemon and vinegar instead, or make the healthy dressings I offer on pages 202–203. In restaurants, ask for dressing on the side and dip your fork into the dressing instead of pouring it over the salad.

Vegetables: As long as they are raw, steamed, or grilled with little or no butter or oil, enjoy them anytime.

LIMITED

Fruit: Bananas and grapes are high in carbs and sugar; keep those to a minimum.

Dried Fruit: It's sugary, but at least it's not added sugar.

Yams: If you roast them long enough they caramelize and don't need butter.

Rice and Potatoes: Do not fry either of these.

Also: Nuts; cheese; sugar-free whipped cream; butter; nonfat, unsweetened yogurt; low-fat cottage cheese.

HIGHLY RESTRICTED

Processed Foods: Frozen dinners, breakfast cereals, instant ramen noodles.

Refined Carbs: Pizza, bread, cake, pastry, doughnuts, pancakes, pasta, candy.

Sugar: Chocolate, candy, ice cream.

Deep-Fried Foods: French fries, fried chicken or fish, mozzarella sticks, egg rolls.

Note: If you like sweets, try xylitol-based candies and Edy's Slow Churned No Sugar Added Ice Cream.

uously. Three issues come to mind with this approach: time, cost, and portion size. Buying food and prepping six meals per day can be a huge money and time investment. And using a meal-delivery service will save time but won't be cheap. Still, even for those who are willing to invest the time and money, if you overdo it with portion sizes, those six small meals can easily turn into four big meals, a medium meal, and a snack.

Choose Whole Grains over Refined Grains

RESEARCHERS AT PENN State University placed 50 obese subjects into two groups. One group was told to eat whole grains as their only grain choices; the other was advised to avoid whole grains. Both groups were asked to do moderate exercise. After 12 weeks, the exercisers who ate whole grains lost a significantly larger percentage of belly fat than those who ate refined grains. Furthermore, their levels of C-reactive protein (CRP), a warning signal of heart disease and diabetes, dropped by 38 percent, while the people who avoided whole-grain foods saw no change in their CRP levels.

Supplement Wisely

FLIP THROUGH MOST fitness magazines and by the time you're finished, you'll likely be convinced that sports supplementation is a must for those who are serious about fitness. Don't believe the hype. I don't take any goofy sports supplements—just what my doctor approves or prescribes: a pill to regulate cholesterol, low-dose baby aspirin, vitamin D in the wintertime, the amino acid citrulline, and whey protein in my shakes for recovery. That's it.

Teamwork multiplies success.

—Cam Goldberg, 32, The Program

For most of Cam's life, fitness was just part of his sports preparation—a tool to drive performance on the football field. Cam played at Duke University and in the NFL briefly. After his football career ended, he carried 75 to 80 pounds of extra weight. ("Still handsome, though," he winks.) With no reason to be huge anymore, Cam had to figure out how to get to his desired shape. When he tried the varied workouts of The Program, he stumbled—he went from being one of the top athletes in the room to one of the more awkward. He also had to stop eating whatever he wanted. When Cam started writing down his fitness goals, things began to change.

In one of his first workouts with The Program, he felt a rush he hadn't felt in years—the feeling of being on a team. A year or so ago, Cam underwent shoulder surgery. Worse than the recovery was sitting on the sidelines watching others keep on crushing it. "No one felt bad for me for one second, and they pushed me to work as hard as possible in physical therapy," Cam says. "I worked around my surgery rather than using it as an excuse and found myself in the best shape of my life. This group provides something I feel we as humans all crave—a supportive team that pushes each other to be the best we can be. I have yet to see someone walk out of a workout and say, 'Man, that really sucked, and I feel worse off for proving to myself that I could work that hard.' It does not happen."

SUPPLEMENTS I TAKE

LOW-DOSE BABY ASPIRIN Taking a daily low-dose aspirin has been shown to prevent heart disease and, according to a study published in the journal *PLOS ONE*, would save more than 900,000 lives of older Americans, save $692 billion in health costs, and improve life expectancy by more than three months over the next 20 years.

VITAMIN D Chronic vitamin D deficiencies increase your risk of developing heart disease, some cancers, osteoporosis, and more. It is estimated that more than a billion people worldwide suffer from low D levels.

CITRULLINE Research has shown that citrulline can help reduce fatigue, improve endurance, and potentially lower blood pressure.

WHEY PROTEIN Whey is a fast-digesting milk protein that improves strength and lean muscle mass. I use it in smoothies (see pages 204–205) but aim to reach my daily protein intake by eating whole foods.

SUPPLEMENTS I DON'T TAKE

CREATINE

There's nothing wrong with creatine—it's been proven to work. However, as it works to help you acquire strength it also creates water retention in your muscles, which can make you look puffy. That's not the look I'm after. Plus, the effects are temporary. As soon as you stop taking it, you lose whatever gains you've made using it.

PRE-WORKOUT ENERGY DRINKS

Some pre-workout drinks label themselves "N.O. boosters," meaning they will increase nitric oxide to promote blood and oxygen flow. They won't. You'll likely feel "pumped up" after drinking one because there's niacin (vitamin B_3) in it, which gives you a flush, making your skin red and warm. Others contain beta-alanine, which produces a harmless but often uncomfortable "pins and needles" feeling and is promoted as an endurance enhancer. Almost all pre-workout energy drinks contain a large dose of caffeine—some as much as 400 mg, the total amount new research suggests you have in a day.

On its own, caffeine offers plenty of benefits: It has been proven to provide a boost of energy and help improve focus, aerobic exercise, and overall power. A study published in the *British Journal of Sports Science* found that subjects who ingested coffee before running 1,500 meters on the treadmill were 4.2 seconds faster on average than those in the control group. Another study published in the *Journal of Strength and Conditioning Research* analyzed nine men who ingested coffee, decaf coffee plus caffeine, caffeine in gel cap form, or a placebo before squatting or bench-pressing. The subjects who ingested coffee and decaffeinated coffee plus caffeine showed improved performance on the squat versus those who took a placebo. This is why I like to have an espresso in the morning before I train. However, drinking just one 32-ounce energy drink can result in "profound changes" to your heart and be particularly harmful to the one in three Americans who have hypertension, according to research published in the *Journal of the American Heart Association*. (See page 115 for more about the benefits of coffee.)

SUPPLEMENTS I DON'T TAKE

STEROIDS

Professional bodybuilders all take steroids. You cannot be or look like a professional bodybuilder without taking steroids. I'm a risk-averse guy who will not put everything on the line for gain, which is why I won't take steroids or unproven, untested supplements or follow extreme diets.

Choosing to take steroids effectively moves your life span forward. You'll be bigger and more muscular and feel more youthful, but there's no free lunch. I spoke to an endocrinologist about this topic, and he said he's seen athletes who supplemented with steroids in their 20s and are now in their 40s and look like they're in their 70s. I'll pass. Hopefully, you'll do the same.

WEIGHT GAINERS

Staying trim typically becomes more challenging as we get older. My metabolism took a very long time to slow, but, ultimately, in my 50s it did. Usually, once you enter your mid- to late 20s, gaining weight is not the issue—keeping it off is. So weight gainers usually aren't necessary.

I have a friend my age who didn't take my word for it. At the time he was skinny-fat: thin but out of shape. He started drinking weight gainer because he wanted to turn his belly into . . . well, I'm not sure what he was looking to do. I suggested that he forgo the weight gainer and instead spend the next 90 days lifting weights and doing low-intensity cardio and high-intensity interval training.

He listened to the info in the magazines, didn't exercise much, and rapidly packed on 25 pounds. He was no longer skinny-fat; he was just fat.

Keeping an open mind can lead to open doors.

—Nate Miller, 30, The Program

Nate stayed fit by playing competitive soccer for 14 years. He moved to New York City after college and quickly packed on 20 pounds. One of his best buddies, Nick Sizer (page 157), told him about The Program, and since he began training with us Nate has become one of the fittest guys in the group.

"I have taken big risks, and while I haven't accomplished everything with flying colors, I have become more confident in myself, leading me to try new things I would have never tried years ago," he says. "Best of all, I have grown into a better person, and that has opened doors that can lead me in any direction I choose to go."

25 Easy Ways to Increase Protein Intake

Protein is extremely important to building lean muscle, which is why each of your three meals in the Becoming Ageless Eating Plan should be protein-centric. But you may find that consuming up to 1 gram per pound of your body weight can be a chore, especially if you rely on the same foods—for example, eggs and grilled chicken—each meal. While whey and plant-based protein powders can help bridge a protein deficiency, those who prefer whole foods can refer to this list of the 25 best natural protein sources.

Plant Protein Sources

ALMONDS

Protein Punch: 6 g per 1 oz, 164 calories

A 24-week study of overweight and obese subjects found that those who ate nuts experienced a 62 percent greater reduction in weight and BMI. For optimal results, eat your daily serving before you train. Almonds, rich in the amino acid L-arginine, can actually help you burn more fat and carbs during workouts, according to a study in *The Journal of the International Society of Sports Nutrition*.

ARTICHOKES

Protein Punch: 4.2 g per 1 medium-size artichoke, 60 calories

Ghrelin is your body's "I'm hungry" hormone, and it's suppressed when your stomach is full, so eating satiating high-fiber and high-protein foods will help to tamp it down. The artichoke is a winner on both counts: It has almost twice as much fiber as kale (10.3 g per medium artichoke, or 40 percent of the daily fiber the average woman needs) and one of the highest protein counts among vegetables. Boil and eat the whole vegetable as a self-contained salad, or toss the leaves with your favorite greens and dressing.

BEANS

Protein Punch: 7 g to 10 g per ½ cup, 109 to 148 calories

Beans are loaded with protein, antioxidants, vitamins, and minerals that can benefit your brain and muscles. They're also slow to digest, which can help you feel fuller, curb hunger cravings, and fuel weight-loss efforts. Look for precooked varieties in BPA-free cans. Add them to soups and salads or mix them with brown rice and steamed vegetables to create a hearty—and healthy—dinner.

CASHEWS

Protein Punch: 5 g per 1 oz, 157 calories

Along with being a quality protein source, cashews also provide you with phosphorus, magnesium, calcium, and copper. Magnesium boasts a myriad of health benefits, such as helping your body relieve various conditions like constipation, insomnia, headaches, and muscle cramps, as well as regulating the immune system and supporting brain function.

CHIA SEEDS

Protein Punch: 5 g per 1 oz, 138 calories

One of the hallmarks of a balanced diet is to have a good ratio of omega-6 fatty acids to omega-3s, which are essential nutrients that aid heart health and brain function, respectively, among other things. A 4-to-1 ratio would be ideal, but the modern American diet is more like 20-to-1. That leads to inflammation, which can cause weight gain. Since eating a serving of salmon every day isn't realistic, sprinkling chia seeds—among the most highly concentrated sources of omega-3s—into smoothies, salads, or even desserts is as easy a diet upgrade as you can get.

LENTILS

Protein Punch: 18 g per 1 cup, 230 calories

One cup of lentils delivers the same amount of protein as three eggs, with less than 1 gram of fat. Their high-fiber content makes them extremely satiating, and studies have shown that eating them can speed fat loss: Spanish researchers found that people whose diets included four weekly servings of legumes lost more weight and improved their cholesterol more than people whose diet didn't. Eat them on their own or as a side or simmer them into a soup.

PEANUT BUTTER

Protein Punch: 7 g per 2 Tbsp, 191 calories

Two tablespoons of peanut butter provide a solid dose of muscle-building protein and 16 grams of healthy fats. According to a 2014 study published in *The American Journal of Clinical Nutrition*, consuming peanuts can prevent both cardiovascular and coronary artery disease— the most common type of heart condition. Select varieties that are unsalted and that contain no added sugar. However, if you're looking to cut back on fat consumption, consider a powdered peanut butter like PB2. Mixing 2 tablespoon of PB2 with 1 tablespoon of water delivers just 45 calories, 1.5 grams of fat, 5 grams of carbs, and 5 grams of protein. Just like peanut butter, it's perfect for smoothies or slathering onto an apple.

PEAS

Protein Punch: 8 g per 1 cup, 118 calories

A cup of green peas contains eight times the protein of a cup of spinach. And with almost 100 percent of your daily value of vitamin C in a single cup, they'll help keep your immune system up to snuff. Layer them into a mason jar salad or add them to an omelet to boost eggs' satiating power.

PUMPKIN SEEDS (SHELLED)

Protein Punch: 9 g per 1 oz, 158 calories

Pumpkin seeds are an excellent source of protein, healthy fats, and fiber, which will help keep you feeling full and energized. Plus, they deliver manganese, magnesium, phosphorus, and zinc, which provide additional energy. Add them to salads and rice dishes or eat them raw.

SPINACH

Protein Punch: 5 g per 1 cup (cooked), 41 calories

Spinach is a great source of not only protein, but also the antioxidant vitamins A and C and heart-healthy folate. One cup of the green superfood has nearly as much protein as a hard-boiled egg—with half the calories. For the best nutritional boost, steam your spinach instead of eating it raw. This cooking method helps retain vitamins and makes it easier for the body to absorb the green's calcium content. Add a handful to soups, omelets, pasta dishes, and veggie stir-fries, or simply steam it and top with pepper, garlic, olive oil, and a squeeze of lemon.

SPROUTED-GRAIN BREAD

Protein Punch: 8 to 12 g per 2 slices, 138 to 220 calories

This nutrient-dense bread is loaded with folate-filled lentils, protein, and good-for-you grains and seeds like barley and millet. To boost the flavor of your slices, make a vegetable sandwich that's overflowing with avocado slices, roasted red peppers, cucumbers, onions, spinach, and tomatoes, and use hummus as your condiment. Limit yourself to two slices.

SUN-DRIED TOMATOES

Protein Punch: 6 g per 1 cup, 139 calories

Tomatoes are packed with the antioxidant lycopene, which studies show can decrease your risk of bladder, lung, prostate, skin, and stomach cancers, as well as reduce the risk of coronary artery disease. Just one of the sun-dried version will give you 6 grams of satiating protein, 7 grams of fiber, and three-fourths of your recommended daily allowance of potassium, which is essential for heart health and tissue repair. They're also rich in vitamins A and K. Use them as a tangy addition to salads or snack on them right out of the bag.

TEFF

Protein Punch: 7 g per ¼ cup, 180 calories

This nutty-flavored gluten-free grain is loaded with fiber, essential amino acids, calcium, and vitamin C—a nutrient not typically found in grains. To reap the benefits, swap your morning oatmeal for a protein-packed teff porridge. In a medium saucepan, combine ½ cup of teff with 1½ cups of water and a pinch of salt. Let it come to a boil before turning the heat down to low and letting it simmer for 15 to 20 minutes. Remove from the heat and top with apples, cinnamon, and some natural peanut butter or PB2.

Animal Protein Sources

BISON
Protein Punch: 23 g per 4 oz, 166 calories

While grass-fed beef is an excellent choice, bison's profile has been rising in recent years, and for good reason: It has half the fat of and fewer calories than red meat. According to the USDA, while a 90 percent lean hamburger may average 10 grams of fat, a comparatively sized buffalo burger rings in at 2 grams of fat with 24 grams of protein, making it one of the leanest meats around. In addition, just one serving delivers a full day's allowance of vitamin B_{12}, which has been shown to boost energy and help shut down the genes responsible for insulin resistance and the formation of fat cells.

CANNED LIGHT TUNA
Protein Punch: 16 g per 3 oz, 73 calories

As a top source of protein and docosahexaenoic acid (DHA), canned light tuna is one of the best and most affordable fish for weight loss and muscle growth. One study in the *Journal of Lipid Research* showed that omega-3 fatty acid supplementation had the profound ability to turn off abdominal fat genes. And while you'll find two types of fatty acids in cold-water fish and fish oils—DHA and eicosapentaenoic acid (EPA)—researchers say DHA can be 40 to 70 percent more effective than EPA at down-regulating fat genes in the abdomen, preventing belly fat cells from expanding in size.

But what about the mercury? Mercury levels in tuna vary by species; generally speaking, the larger and leaner the fish, the higher the mercury level. Bluefin and albacore rank among the most toxic, according to a study in *Biology Letters*. But canned chunk light tuna, harvested from the smallest fish, is considered a "low-mercury fish" and can be enjoyed two to three times a week (or up to 12 ounces), according to the FDA.

Lastly, opt for tuna packed in water, which contains fewer calories and less saturated fat than oil-packed tuna.

CHICKEN

Protein Punch: 26 g per 3-oz breast (cooked), 142 calories

A 3-ounce cooked chicken breast contains only 142 calories and 3 grams of fat but packs a whopping 26 grams of protein.

EGGS

Protein Punch: 7 g per 1 egg, 85 calories

Eggs might just be the easiest, cheapest, and most versatile way to increase your protein intake. Each 85-calorie egg packs a solid 7 grams of the muscle builder and is loaded with amino acids, antioxidants, and iron.

Don't discard the yolks, either. Egg yolk contains a fat-fighting nutrient called choline, so opting for whole eggs can actually help you trim down. When you're shopping for eggs, pay attention to the labels. Buy organic when possible. These eggs are certified by the USDA and are free from antibiotics, vaccines, and hormones.

GRASS-FED BEEF

Protein Punch: 26 g per 4-oz strip steak, 133 calories

Grass-fed steak and burgers are more expensive, but grass-fed beef is naturally leaner and has fewer calories than conventional meat: A lean 7-ounce conventional strip steak has 386 calories and 16 grams of fat. But a 7-ounce grass-fed strip steak has only 233 calories and 5 grams of fat. According to a study published in *Nutrition Journal,* grass-fed meat also contains higher levels of omega-3 fatty acids, which have been shown to reduce the risk of heart disease.

GREEK YOGURT (NONFAT, PLAIN)
Protein Punch: 20 g per 7 oz, 150 calories

Yogurt may be one of your key allies in weight-loss efforts. A study in the *Journal of Nutrition* found that probiotics in yogurt helped obese women lose nearly twice the weight compared with those who did not consume probiotics. Both sets of subjects were on low-calorie diets, but after 12 weeks, the probiotic group lost an average of 9.7 pounds, while those on placebos lost only 5.7.

GROUND TURKEY
Protein Punch: 16 g per 4-oz turkey burger, 140 calories

Lean and protein-rich, a quarter-pound turkey burger patty contains 140 calories, 16 grams of protein, and 8 grams of fat. Additionally, turkey is rich in DHA omega-3 acids—18 milligrams per serving, the highest on this list—which has been shown to boost brain function, improve your mood, and prevent fat cells from growing. Stick with white meat; dark meat contains too much fat.

GRUYÈRE CHEESE
Protein Punch: 8 g per 1 oz, 117 calories

One slice of this Swiss cheese contains 30 percent more protein than an egg, plus one-third of your RDA of vitamin A. When indulging, keep your serving to the size of four dice.

HALIBUT
Protein Punch: 16 g per 3 oz, 77 calories

You might be surprised to learn that halibut tops fiber-rich oatmeal and vegetables in the satiety department. The Satiety Index of Common Foods, an Australian study published in the *European Journal of Clinical Nutrition*, ranks it the No. 2 most filling food—bested only by boiled potatoes. A separate Australian study that compared the satiety of different animal proteins found a nutritionally similar white fish to be significantly more satiating than beef and chicken; satiety following the white fish meal also declined at a much slower rate. Study authors attribute the filling factor of white fish like halibut to its impressive protein content.

OSTRICH

Protein Punch: 29 g per 4-oz patty, 194 calories

Ostrich meat is the rising star of the grill. While it's technically a red meat and has the rich taste of beef, ostrich has less fat than turkey or chicken. A 4-ounce patty contains nearly 30 grams of muscle-building protein and just 6 grams of fat. A nutritional bonus: One serving has 200 percent of the recommended daily allowance of vitamin B_{12}. This exotic increasingly popular entrée also contains 55 milligrams of choline, one of the essential nutrients for fat loss.

PORK

Protein Punch: 24 g per 4 oz, 124 calories

Lately, pork has been recognized as healthier than previously thought, so long as you choose the right cut. Stick with pork tenderloin: A University of Wisconsin study found that a 3-ounce serving of pork tenderloin has slightly less fat than a skinless chicken breast. It has 24 grams of protein per serving and 83 milligrams of choline (about the same as a medium egg). In a study published in the journal *Nutrients*, scientists asked 144 overweight people to eat a diet rich in fresh lean pork. After three months, the group saw a significant reduction in waist size, BMI, and belly fat, with no reduction in muscle mass. The scientists speculate that the amino acid profile of pork protein may contribute to greater fat burning.

WILD SALMON

Protein Punch: 17 g per 3 oz, 121 calories

Don't let salmon's relatively high calorie and fat content fool you; research suggests that the oily fish may be one of the best for weight loss. In one study, participants were divided into groups and assigned one of three equicaloric weight-loss diets: one that had no seafood (the control group), one that included lean white fish, or one that included salmon. Everyone lost weight, but the salmon eaters had the lowest fasting insulin levels and a marked reduction in inflammation. Another study in the *International Journal of Obesity* found that eating three 5-ounce servings of salmon per week for four weeks as part of a low-calorie diet resulted in approximately 2.2 pounds more weight lost than following an equicaloric diet that didn't include fish. Wild salmon is leaner than farmed salmon, which is plumped up on fish meal, and it's also proven to be significantly lower in cancer-linked PCBs.

CHAPTER 5

Break
the Glass

The path to a cleaner and healthier lifestyle requires the right drinks in the right amounts at the right times. Follow this crystal-clear guide to perfect hydration.

IT'S EASY TO overlook the caloric danger that comes from what we drink—not eat. In one sitting you can quickly slurp, sip, or guzzle hundreds (and in some cases, thousands) of calories in all kinds of forms. The fancy coffee drink you have twice a day may be more like a milkshake. (And the milkshake you have could be the caloric equivalent of an entire day's meals.) Sodas and sports drinks contain too much sugar. The American Heart Association recommends an upper limit of just 36 grams of sugar per day. An easy way to blow through that is to drink one

12-ounce can of soda, which has 39 grams of sugar. Orange juice? Too much sugar there, too. And then there's beer, wine, and cocktails. The problem is that liquid calories all go down so fast, you hardly notice them. And it's not like you even enjoyed them all that much.

When I was in graduate school at Harvard getting my MBA and law degrees, I found myself with a lot of free time on my hands. (Trust me: Studying two subjects is a lot easier than studying seven, like an undergrad.) One particular evening, I met a few friends at my buddy Ted's apartment. It was a typical student apartment—dimly lit, minimal furniture, dishes that needed to be cleaned, and floors that could have used a mop—and we were doing what all college kids do in their downtime: drinking beer. Though I don't recall every fine detail of this evening—it was almost 40 years ago, after all—I remember this conversation vividly:

"Dude, you have a paunch," Ted said to me while pointing to my stomach.

I looked at my midsection and studied it for a moment. Admittedly, diet and exercise weren't of great concern at the time, but me with a paunch? No way, Ted. "No, I don't. I'm skinny!" I replied.

He persisted. "No, no—you say that you're skinny, but you *actually* have a paunch. You. Have. A. Paunch!"

He was right. The combo of not exercising and not paying attention to what I ate had caught up with me.

The conversation prompted me to take action—I began a body-weight workout the following day—but also demonstrated the fact that to build a lean and healthy body required taking a realistic look at not only what I was putting on my plate but also what was being poured into my glass. Frankly, it should be nothing more than water. Staying hydrated with pure water benefits your health, energy level, and body composition. Pretty much every other drink has some negative

4 WAYS TO DRINK MORE WATER

Here's the smoothest way to make the switch once you decide to drop your high-calorie drinks for water:

1) Drink two glasses when you wake up, two glasses before every meal, and then one glass before bed. This gives you a routine to follow so that you're matching one action (like waking up), with a trigger to take another action (having two glasses).

2) Give yourself a daily goal—say, 12 eight-ounce glasses of water. (Or go up to a full gallon if you're up for it.) Commit to two weeks of making sure you get this amount.

3) If you have a sweet tooth, add flavor to water by adding slices of fruit or a natural sweetener like xylitol, a sugar alcohol that looks and tastes like sugar but doesn't raise blood sugar levels.

4) If you have trouble hitting the daily allotment, try keeping a glass on your desk; you'll naturally sip at it as your body looks for breaks from the screen, assuming you work in that kind of environment.

component and therefore should be consumed in limited quantities or eliminated.

We used to think drinking eight 8-ounce cups of water per day was ideal to remain hydrated. The Institute of Medicine now suggests at least 11 cups per day for women and 15 for men. I recommend drinking 16 ounces of water when you wake up, with meals, before bed, and whenever you feel thirsty.

This new habit will pay off. A study from the University of Illinois published in the *Journal of Human Nutrition and Dietetics* examined the dietary habits of more than 18,300 U.S. adults. The study examined data from the National Health and Nutrition Examination Survey, which was conducted by the National Center for Health Statistics. It found that the majority of people who increased their consumption of plain water (tap water or from a cooler, drinking fountain, or bottle) by 1 percent reduced their total daily calorie intake as well as their consumption of saturated fat, sugar, sodium, and cholesterol. People who increased their consumption of water by one, two, or three cups daily decreased their total energy intake by 68 to 205 calories daily and their sodium intake by 78 to 235 milligrams. They also consumed 5 grams to nearly 18 grams less sugar and decreased their cholesterol consumption by 7 to 21 milligrams daily. (The impact of plain water intake on diet was similar across race/ethnicity, education and income levels, and body-weight status.)

Drinking two glasses of water before you eat is another smart strategy. That helps fill you up, so you're less likely to eat a lot at your meal. (It takes some 20 minutes for your brain to realize that you're satisfied, which is one of the reasons why we overeat: We eat too quickly.)

A study conducted by researchers from the University of Birmingham in the U.K. and published in the journal *Obesity* sought to determine the effectiveness of water preloading before meals as a weight-loss strategy. Eighty-four obese adults were given a face-to-face weight-management consultation at baseline and a follow-up telephone consultation at two weeks. Participants were randomized to either drinking 16 ounces of water 30 minutes before their main meals or being part of an attention-control group that asked them to imagine their stomach was already full before meals. Weight change was recorded at the 12-week follow-up. Those who drank water before each main meal lost an average of 9.5 pounds. Drinking water before just one meal per day led to an average weight loss of 1.76 pounds.

Another study, this one out of Virginia Tech, looked at a similar question. The small study divided subjects into two groups. One group drank two cups of water prior to meals, and the other did not. All the subjects ate a low-calorie diet during the study. Over the course of 12 weeks, the water drinkers lost about 15.5 pounds, while the non-water drinkers lost about 11 pounds. The theory as to why water is so effective is simple: It fills up the stomach with a substance that has zero calories.

I know that it can be a challenge to make a full-blown switch to something that "tastes like nothing" if you're used to drinking juice, soda, or other sweetened drinks. So I'm not saying that the first few weeks will be seamless, but you can take some measures to help retrain your taste buds and establish a new habit. For example, you can flavor your water by adding slices of fruit or vegetables. Lemons and limes work well, but some people use apples, grapes, or even cucumbers.

Coffee and Tea

THESE TWO FAVORITES are among the most widely sipped beverages worldwide. More than half of the U.S. population age 50 and over consumes coffee daily. Both drinks can provide health benefits like reduced risk of stroke, coronary heart disease, type 2 diabetes, and Parkinson's disease. However, adding sugar and milk or cream can increase calories and promote fat storage. (Some flavored coffees at coffee shops like Dunkin' Donuts and Starbucks contain more than 45 grams of sugar.) If you want a sweetener, use xylitol and a little skim milk.

◆ **Coffee might offset the adverse effects of obesity**
A University of Georgia study found that chlorogenic acid (CGA), a chemical compound found in coffee, could potentially prevent some of the damaging effects of obesity, including increased insulin resistance and liver steatosis (or the accumulation of fat in the liver).

◆ **Coffee can boost exercise endurance**
A study in the *International Journal of Sport Nutrition and Exercise Metabolism* sought to evaluate the effects of pre-exercise coffee on athletes' endurance and exertion. Looking

at the nine trials, the authors concluded that between 3 and 7 milligrams of caffeine per kilogram of body weight increased exercise endurance by an average of 24 percent.

◆ **Green tea consumption has links to weight loss**
In some studies, green tea has been shown to support weight loss, lower total cholesterol, raise HDL (good) cholesterol, and reduce inflammation associated with inflammatory bowel disease (aka IBD).

Alcohol

SOME EVIDENCE SUGGESTS that moderate alcohol consumption can provide minor cardiovascular benefits, including helping prevent heart disease and stroke. However, alcohol metabolizes to sugar, yielding empty calories and hindering muscle growth and fat loss. It doesn't make a lot of sense to train hard and adopt a healthier diet only to sabotage your results with the wrong kind of six-pack. Additionally, alcohol is a depressant that slows down vital bodily functions and can lower inhibitions, which can lead to more unplanned cheat meals and higher caloric intake.

As it happens, I don't drink anymore. About six years ago I gave it up to rid my body of toxins in order to focus on living a healthier, stronger life. The decision wasn't easy to make because I liked Scotch, but I was also consuming two drinks—and a few hundred extra calories—each night. If I was going to wake up at 5 a.m. and get superfit, the alcohol had to go. I had no choice.

Ultimately, it was the right thing to do. The effects—both physical and emotional—have been amazing. But that choice is certainly not for everyone, and moderate drinking can be just fine. If you do drink, choose a low-carb spirit, like vodka, without sugary mixers such as soda or juice. Also, on a night out, begin and end your evening with water.

Milk and Juice

WE HAVE TRADITIONALLY been told that both milk and juice are good for us. In fact, I was brought up believing that a healthy breakfast had to include both. More recent research calls that into question.

It's not that these drinks don't have some redeeming value. Calcium is indeed good for bone strength, and 100 percent fruit juice does include disease-fighting compounds. The problem is, a good ingredient does not necessarily make for a healthy food.

I don't drink juice; it has little or no fiber and is primarily composed of fructose (aka sugar). I prefer to get the benefits from fruit in its natural form, which include fiber.

And as for milk, I don't want the added calories, fat, and sugar. I get my protein in other, healthier forms, such as eggs, chicken breast, and fish. And I get calcium through leafy greens and other forms of dairy, such as yogurt and cheese. I do have milk or half-and-half in my coffee. Whole milk is caloric, though, and skim milk is carby, so don't overdo it.

The research is mixed on the correlation between consuming dairy products and weight gain. Some studies show a positive association between consuming dairy products and lower obesity. On the other hand, a Tufts University study published in the *American Journal of Clinical Nutrition* followed 51,529 males from all 50 states and found that consumption of low-fat dairy products actually promotes weight gain. Researchers suggested that the subjects compensated for the lower caloric content of low-fat dairy by increasing their intake of other carbs and calories.

And when it comes to juice, a Harvard University study tracked the dietary and lifestyle habits of more than 120,000 men and women over a 20-year span. Based on data from the study showing a correlation, researchers determined that fruit juice consumption led to weight gain.

Push your limits.

—Katie Tuttle, 31, The Program

G rowing up, Katie didn't play traditional sports, but she did develop an appreciation for movement, form, and technique through dance. A friend dragged her to her first hot power yoga class in 2011. Though she thought the 105-degree room was stifling and found the heavy breathing annoying, she was soon practicing daily.

"I felt connected to something bigger than myself. My body got stronger and my mind more focused," Katie says. "It was the catalyst of this amazing journey of self-discovery through fitness that I've been loving and living ever since."

Katie expanded her fitness interests to include barre, Pilates, weight training, CrossFit, and powerlifting.

"I mean, really, is there anything more empowering than having a barbell loaded with more than my body weight on my back or deadlifting twice my body weight?" she asks.

Through fitness, she's learned that she craves challenges and testing her limits. When she joined The Program, her passions intensified.

"This team has given me purpose," she says. "They are my teachers, mentors, motivators, and, most of all, my family. We aren't perfect. Sometimes we fail. But this team shows up for one another. We elevate each other. It's just what we do and who we are. Period."

CHAPTER 6

Cheat Like a Champ

Maximize your results and motivation by intelligently indulging in your favorite foods.

UNQUESTIONABLY, if the only foods I ate were steamed broccoli and chicken breast I would be leaner. But I'd also be miserable, and that's no way for anyone to walk through life. Though I've figured out a cheat schedule that suits my needs, sticking to it is an ongoing exercise in self-discipline. One story comes to mind that embodies something I go through fairly often: I met a friend for breakfast at a restaurant known for having the most delicious, mouthwatering ricotta cheese pancakes. As I scanned the menu, I had an urge to order them. *Treat yourself,* I thought. *You already worked out this* *morning, so you can afford the extra calories.* I was close to pulling the trigger on the pancakes—until I remembered the handful of french fries I ate the night before. The serving size was moderate, but that didn't make it any less of a cheat. Then I looked at my schedule and realized that an early-afternoon meeting would likely cause me to miss lunch. Lastly, there was my list of "wants." I couldn't justify the excess calories.

No, turning down pancakes wasn't a life-changing decision, but for those of you who enjoy sweets and cheats, I understand how much of a struggle it can be to stay strong. When you're feeling weak, remind yourself of the goals you wrote down and understand that caving too many times will make achieving them even more of an uphill battle. But staying the course does require sacrifice to obtain the body and life you want. When I do allow myself treats, I try hard not to overdo it. As Dr. Attia, my doctor and consultant on food's effects on longevity, has told me, my cheat days are probably better than many people's good days.

However, what I won't do is put myself on a totally restrictive diet. If people tell you they eat a certain way all the time—just greens with no oil or dressing and raw fruits and vegetables, for example—they're probably not telling the truth.

Keeping that in mind, I still don't limit the cheat foods I eat, because I know that denying myself a food I want only increases the odds that I will turn to it when a hunger craving strikes. However, if you are unable to use moderation with certain foods, consider removing them from the "highly restricted" category and creating another category titled "never."

The Case for Cheat Foods

YOUR BRAIN IS a complex and nuanced system that balances both emotion and logic. Decisions can be based on emotion. When you're stressed or tired, a jolt of glucose into your

Skip dessert.

—Roland Hernandez, 60, The Program

Roland was my roommate in law school. He played tennis in high school and squash in college and became an avid runner and cyclist after earning his law degree. Work often keeps him on the road and prevents him from training with The Program, but he engages in plenty of rigorous cross-training to compete in his latest passion: triathlons.

"I'm 5-foot-11 and 156 pounds—the same weight and waist size I was in high school," he says.

Something that helped get him there: passing on desserts.

"I don't find desserts to be necessary. If I put on an extra three pounds, I am going to pay for it when I race," he says.

---

bloodstream triggers a dopamine response that leads to a short-term boost in energy, mood, and productivity. When dopamine levels subside, your body seeks to elevate them again. Sugar and simple carbs can do that quickly, but you will eventually need more and more to keep dopamine levels elevated. And the cycle continues at the expense of your waistline.

While some experts strongly suggest complete elimination of cheat foods, I think it's facile to tell you to stop eating them and to stop eating with emotion. Deprivation can also be a negative and powerful force. For some people it's possible to avoid entirely foods that are bad for them. For others, trying too hard to do so will yield an opposite effect: We reach a point at which we simply abandon a healthy diet altogether.

The goal is to find that delicate balance between exercising healthy willpower, eating strategically, and training oneself to be satisfied with less.

How to Cheat Intelligently

CHEAT FOODS FALL into the following main categories: ultra-processed foods, refined carbs, and sugar. Being sensible about cheating can help keep your diet on point. So build it into your overall meal plan using one these strategies:

- **Cheat on one assigned day per week, as long as you eat nearly perfectly the other six.**
- **Adopt a four-days-on (clean), one-day-off (cheat) plan. I have found this method to be the most effective for me.**
- **Cheat a little each day.**

Whichever approach you take, the key is to manage portions—fill a mug with ice cream instead of a bowl, for example.

Write It Down

DR. ATTIA'S SPECIALTY is nutrition's effect on longevity, which is originally why I sought him out. At the time, I was an unusual patient for him because I wasn't elderly, sick, or overweight. I just wanted to live a healthier life. Still, he agreed to see me, and our first consultation went something like this: "I don't drink, smoke, or use drugs. I'm not overweight. I'm fit, I train hard, and I eat a balanced diet that includes sweets. My diet is not up for discussion."

I *really* didn't want to give up my junk-food habit. I cherished cakes, candy, chips—everything. And to his credit, Dr. Attia didn't push me. Months later, he suggested that I keep a food diary to keep tabs on what I was consuming on a daily basis. I thought it was a fair request, and for two weeks I was diligent about recording everything I put into my body. I had no idea how impactful the exercise in food journaling would be, but studies have found that it's a vastly effective way to increase weight loss:

◆ **Keeping a daily food journal can double weight-loss efforts**
A six-month study conducted by Kaiser Permanente found that people who kept a daily food journal lost 18 pounds, versus nine pounds for those who didn't log their food intake regularly. In a separate study that appeared in the *Journal of the Academy of Nutrition and Dietetics*, subjects who kept accurate food journals lost about six pounds more than subjects who didn't over a one-year period.

◆ **Self-monitoring food intake heightens dietary awareness**
Participants who were asked to recall their last meal before doing a taste test ate 30 percent fewer cookies than those who were asked about their morning commute, according to a study published in the journal *Physiology & Behavior*. Researchers believe that knowing and remembering what you ate triggers your brain's hippocampus, which potentially helps you refrain from consuming extra calories.

When I reviewed my food journal, I discovered that my meals were nutritionally balanced, but upon closer examination, it was clear that my snacking habit needed to be tamed. In the moment, you don't think that eating one or two peanut butter cups, a handful of M&M's, or a scoop of ice cream will have much of an impact. Individually, they might not. Collectively, they can and do. It became clear that changes to my diet were not negotiable if I was to follow through with my fitness goals.

Show up, don't give up.

—Jessica Lippke, 34, The Program

Jessica grew up playing volleyball, basketball, and lacrosse, ultimately playing Division I volleyball at Hofstra University. After college, she discovered CrossFit and fell in love with its community and philosophy. Eventually, her drive and passion for CrossFit waned, and she spent a year struggling to find her new fitness home, gaining more than 30 pounds along the way. For her 30th birthday, she asked her husband for a barbell and plates to start doing at-home workouts and lifts. While it filled the void, she missed the group atmosphere. Jessica's memories and life lessons have come from being part of a team. Within six months of joining The Program, she lost 35 pounds and reignited her passion for health and fitness. She credits The Program's balance of fitness, mindfulness, nutrition, and goal setting for much of her success.

"There are few things worth waking up at 4:30 a.m. for—a workout with The Program is one of them. When you have a team of people, all different ages, all different backgrounds, and on different career paths, but all with a common mind-set, waiting for you to walk in the door in the morning, you don't want to let them down. You show up. Everyone has their own story, and I'm really happy The Program is part of mine."

It's not uncommon for many of us to eat without being aware of calorie content. And eating while being distracted—watching television, for instance—increases calorie intake. So a food journal through an app, a spreadsheet, or a notepad will help you identify eating patterns and improve your behavior. Once you know exactly what you're eating and see in black and white the associated caloric effects, you'll be motivated to make adjustments. (That's the start of an ageless eating plan like the one on pages 178–179.)

Of course, there are plenty of apps that make it easy for you to track your food intake. I like FatSecret (fatsecret.com). Other popular options include My Macros+ (getmymacros.com), Fitocracy (fitocracy.com), and MyFitnessPal (myfitnesspal.com). Monitoring enables you to recognize patterns and identify areas where you're most vulnerable.

Change Your Language

INSTEAD OF SAYING you "can't," try saying you "don't." This subtle change shifts the power from a rule to a choice. Research published in the *Journal of Consumer Research* divided students into two groups: One group was told that when faced with a specific temptation, they should tell themselves "I can't." The second group was told to say "I don't." As each student walked out of the room they handed in their answer sheet and were offered a treat—either a chocolate bar or a health bar. The "I can't" participants ate the chocolate 61 percent of the time, while the "I don't" students chose chocolate only 36 percent of the time. The conclusion was that using the "don't" refusal is more empowering and more likely to lead to resistance to temptation than the "can't" refusal.

This suggests a new way of thinking about the cheat foods that are the most appealing to you: Take them out of the restriction mind-set and make the decision yours.

A BEGINNER'S GUIDE
TO NUTRITION

STEP 1:   Eat three times a day. Regulate your snacking. Start a food diary and write down everything you eat and drink for at least one full week.

STEP 2:   Pick two days a week when you will not have anything from a box or bag. Refer to the *Becoming Ageless Diet Principles* on page 92 and follow them as closely as possible.

STEP 3:   Increase your "good" days from two to three.

WHAT'S NEXT: You're aiming to get to the point at which your diet revolves around my main principles. I like to eat clean four days and then cheat one day, so I work in a five-day cycle rather than a seven-day cycle. Adjust that for your lifestyle so you're not overhauling your diet on Monday just to crash again on Saturday.

Gently eliminate the foods that are more destructive and add the ones that are good for you. It will likely take you at least a month to do so, but don't beat yourself up if it takes two or three months. Chip away at these eating habits and you will get there.

Part Three

BULLETPROOF YOUR BODY

How to prevent illness and disease and stay healthy—forever

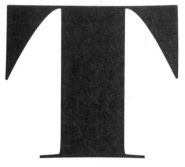**HE FIRST SIX** chapters of the book focused on getting fit and lean. That's a great start. Food and movement are the main variables in the equation. But it would be misleading only to focus on calisthenics and kale. This section expands the discussion to include preservation, diagnostics, and appearance, which together work to promote a healthier body and mind.

The reality is that you're blessed with far more healing power than you may be aware of. In my opinion, our society relies far too much on medicine and quick fixes, and we need to understand that not everything can be fixed with a pill. While medication plays a crucial role in curing illness, I'd argue that we should strive toward another, smarter goal: not getting sick in the first place.

I don't get sick often. Maybe once a year, I'll come down with a cold or the flu, and I think the infrequency has more to do with my lifestyle than genetics or luck. Practicing smart overall health strategies will go a long way in fending off sickness and disease.

Diagnostics, if utilized, are incredibly helpful in identifying, addressing, and avoiding serious medical issues. Too many people ignore warning signs, don't schedule regular appointments, or just think, "It's not going to happen to me." That's a big mistake. We have great technology that's getting more advanced every day. What we don't have is a collective mind-set to maximize these health options.

Finally, how you look matters. I will briefly cover grooming because your appearance forms an important part of the psychology and emotion of good and youthful living.

So in the following section, I want you to think about these areas as ways in which to complement your retooled diet and exercise plans. When you put them all together, you've just about figured out how to take a holistic approach to improving your body inside and out.

CHAPTER 7

Your Health-Preservation Measures

Enlist all the health-minded preventive measures you can today to ensure you're in top form tomorrow and beyond.

AT THE BEGINNING of the book, I asked you to imagine yourself in old age. And now I'd like you to repeat this exercise, only with a subtle tweak: Imagine a watercolor painting of your life 10 or 20 years from now. Why a watercolor? Well, because the details aren't as important as the general sense of where you are as a person. Ask yourself: Are you married? Do you have children? What is your job, or have you retired? Where do you live? How do you live? Is money a factor in your happiness equation? How much leisure time do you have? How do you devote that leisure time?

I painted that watercolor when I was in my teens and my 20s, and more or less, it's where I am now. Getting to this point called for me to make many adjustments to my daily routine, but if I keep this up, in the absence of a horrible injury or illness, I don't see any limitation. Success is really about what you want, and the watercolor helped me create a mental picture of what I envisioned "success" to be.

In my case, my values almost never changed, but they did evolve. Early on, I envisioned running a movie studio and being successful in a more traditional sense, such as financially and in having a family. Over time I revised the painting to give it broader business ambitions and less of a focus on purely financial ones. I realized that after a certain point of success, more financial ambition is really about ego rather than practical use. Now, this in no way implies that I have taken an oath of poverty or that I live a humble existence. I don't—nor do I want to. It's simply that my watercolor evolved to have fewer dollar signs and a greater emphasis on the nature of my relationships with my wife, kids, friends, and colleagues. And as even more time passed, those colors became more specific and saturated to include an array of digitally focused media businesses, as well as a focus on service to others professionally, personally, and charitably, along with being engaged in health and wellness and fitness in a fun and meaningful way.

Your goals and aspirations may differ wildly from mine, and that's just fine. But I think it's safe to say that nobody would paint themselves as too obese to bend over and tie their shoes. In the long run, it's easier to make adjustments in how you live now than to deal later with the consequences of not making them. For example, isn't exercising daily better than having heart surgery? Part of the trick is changing your mind-set: What may feel difficult now is vastly better for you in the future.

What I am recommending is delaying gratification—something that adults need to be able to do. In the same way that you save for retirement without questioning it, you need to make healthier life choices now to avoid sickness and decline later on.

I don't want to inundate you with an extensive list of disease-prevention measures. Instead, I'll focus on a few important ones that are doable and necessary if you want to commit to a healthy and strong life.

The Power of Sleep

WHEN I'M STRESSED out I sometimes have difficulties *staying* asleep, but falling asleep isn't usually a problem for me—especially since most of my days begin at 5 a.m. Still, that doesn't make me immune from persuading myself to stay up a little bit later despite knowing that going to bed would be the best thing to do. For some reason, at the time, passing on sleep to watch one more episode of your favorite show, to send one more email, to finish a project, or to have one last drink with your buddies trumps common sense.

> "That's the culture we live in: We're über-connected, we fear missing out, and we want to do more, work more, see more."

I know a lot of people who pride themselves on not needing much sleep and others who say, "I'll sleep when I'm dead." That's the culture we live in: We're über-connected, we fear missing out, and we want to do more, work more, see more. In doing so, we sacrifice sleep—one of the most important elements when it comes to preserving our health.

Show your strength by lifting others up.

—Billy Raiford, 21, The Program

During high school, Billy played football and bulked up to 205 pounds. Following a low-carb diet that omitted processed foods helped him drop down to 160 pounds. And training with The Program helped him reshape his view of just how beneficial exercise can be.

"Before I worked out with The Program I almost always trained alone," he says. "I've found that making fitness a social experience has made it more fun and rewarding. I always thought seeing self-improvement in the mirror was the most rewarding part of the fitness journey, but watching people you care about improve themselves along with you is a much more gratifying and valuable experience.

Sleep deprivation affects nearly half of America's population. In fact, the Centers for Disease Control and Prevention has labeled chronic tiredness a public health problem. The Institute of Medicine estimates that between 50 million and 70 million people suffer from sleep disorders or deprivation, and nearly 9 million Americans take prescription medicine to combat sleeplessness. Now, relying on a sleep aid every so often won't do you much harm. It's when doing so becomes habit that health concerns arise, including diminished REM sleep, memory, attention span, and ability to learn, a University of California San Diego study found.

Additionally, research published in *The American Journal of Public Health* reported that sleep drugs like Ambien and Restoril had the potential to increase meaningfully a driver's risk of getting into an accident. Healthy habits like those in your *Becoming Ageless* eating and workout plans can make it easier to get a good night's sleep and reap the many benefits of quality slumber. Here are some of the ways sleep can make you stronger:

Sleep Supports Weight-Loss Efforts

PEOPLE WHO SLEEP four hours per night eat up to 300 more calories in a day than people who get nine hours of shut-eye per night, according to a Columbia University study. Another study connected sleep deprivation to junk-food binges. Increased consumption of fat, notably saturated fat, was seen in short-span sleepers.

Sleep Improves Learning and Memory

SLEEP DEPRIVATION COMPROMISES one's ability to focus. Also, during sleep, your brain takes what you learned from the previous day and files it away for later use. Depriving your brain of that time can impede those filing and recall efforts. People who sleep immediately after learning perform better on recall tests, according to a study conducted by researchers from the University of Notre Dame.

Sleep Helps Keep Blood Pressure in Check

AVERAGING LESS THAN seven hours of sleep per night was shown to have a direct connection to hypertension in nearly 6,000 human subjects age 40 to 100 years old, according to results from the Sleep Heart Health Study that were published in the journal *Sleep*.

Attitude is everything.

—Sarah Denby, 33, The Program

Sarah was invited to our 6 a.m. cycling class. Her response to the early start time: laughter. But a little persuasion got her to agree to come one morning. When the time came, she overslept. The next week, Sarah tried again and made it—and she was glad she did. Though she was a regular gymgoer, The Program was different.

"Everyone was shouting, cheering, and high-fiving," she says. "I had never worked harder or had more fun."

It's been a few years, and Sarah has changed—she gets up early and has taken her fitness to a new level.

"I've learned to remain positive and not to give up when things don't work out right away. By surrounding myself with such an encouraging crew, I see myself differently. I see people in my life differently, too. I appreciate those who support me, and I've become a much better friend in return. My journey started with a schedule change and resulted in a life change."

Sleep Aids Immune System Function

SUBJECTS IN A Carnegie Mellon University study were quarantined and given nasal drops containing rhinovirus (the main cause of the common cold). Subjects who slept less than seven hours were three times more likely to develop a cold than subjects who slept eight hours. Those with greater sleep efficiency—the total sleep time divided by the total time spent in bed—had even better odds of warding off illness.

Sleep Supports Cancer Prevention

CANCER RESEARCHERS FROM the University of Chicago separated mice into two groups: a group allowed to sleep regularly and a group that was awakened at two-minute intervals during times they normally slept. A week later, all the mice were injected with tumorous cells. All mice developed tumors within two weeks, but the sleep-deprived group's tumors grew twice as large as those in the well-rested group.

If you have trouble sleeping, here are a handful of things I have done or tried to promote a better sleeping environment or more peaceful rest:

1) **Make the room cooler**
   Studies show that a drop in core temperature sends a signal to the body alerting it to power down.

2) **Make the room dark**
   Exposure even to dim light can throw off your circadian rhythm, or what is commonly referred to as your body's biological clock.

3) **Shut down electronic devices an hour before bed**
   The blue light emitted by tablets, computers, smartphones, and other devices has been shown to be particularly disruptive to sleep.

4) **Use your bed for sex and sleep only**
   Read, eat, watch television, and work elsewhere.

5) **Drown out ambient noise**
   Use a fan, noise machine, or smartphone app.

6) **Stretch**
   Try 10 minutes of light stretching before bed.

Have faith in yourself.

—Lainie Goldstein, 50, The Program

After struggling to manage her weight for most of her adult life, Lainie hired a personal trainer and made a commitment to change. After 11 months of hard work and dedication she dropped 90 pounds and 20 percent body fat.

"There have been times when my weight has slowly crept up again," she says. "In the past, I would feel like a failure and just give up. My trainer had faith in me and would not allow that to happen—that was highly motivating. The ability to refocus and get the weight back off is a huge change from the person I used to be."

7) Meditate

Studies show meditation can support relaxation efforts.

8) Think about what's causing your sleeplessness

Try to find the cause. If it's chronic pain or depression—two common sleep disrupters—seek the help of a qualified professional.

The Importance of Water

I DRINK PLENTY of water because of my demanding training schedule. In Chapter 5, I discussed why and how that benefits me and the reason water is a staple in a healthy diet. But water doesn't help only to reduce calorie intake. In addition to keeping

A healthy diet rich in tomatoes, olive oil, nuts, green leafy vegetables, yams, fatty fish, and fruits—along with proper hydration, a strength-driven exercise routine, and quality sleep—can help keep sickness at bay. Use these science-driven methods to help reduce your risk of illness even more.

1) **Wash your hands.** Use soap and water and scrub for at least 20 to 30 seconds.

2) **Filter the air.** High-efficiency particulate air (HEPA) filters can remove nearly 98 percent of virus particles. Pointing a fan out the window can also help.

3) **Train your mind.** People over the age of 50 who underwent mindfulness training, such as meditation, in a University of Wisconsin study nearly halved the occurrence and severity of acute respiratory infections.

you feeling full, it supports normal muscle and organ function, aids skin health and appearance, and enhances energy. Drinking lots of water may very well be the simplest thing you can do to improve your health, and the best part is that it requires minimal effort. I don't believe you necessarily need to drink a set amount of water every day, although more is almost certainly better. As I've mentioned, I recommend consuming 16 ounces first thing in the morning, with meals, before bed, and anytime you get thirsty. In any case, the primary goal is to eliminate unhealthy beverages, including soda, juices, and high-calorie coffee drinks.

If you do nothing else tomorrow as you embark on your journey to live a stronger, healthier life, you can do this.

Stress Reduction

AT THIS POINT in my life, I have more or less learned to manage stress. I generally get enough rest, exercise often, eat a clean

The best diets complement your lifestyle.

—Michael Berland, 50, The Program

Before he wrote the book *Become a Fat-Burning Machine*, Michael was an overweight man in his 40s. At 250 pounds, he knew he needed to make a change. He switched to a diet that featured more fat, fewer carbs, and plenty of protein. Today, Michael has virtually eliminated all processed foods and sugar. After dropping more than 60 pounds, he participated in an Ironman race. "If you don't like being on a diet, then you're not doing it right," he says.

diet, and do my best to not bring work issues home with me. But it's important to remember that all stress isn't bad. For instance, the stress you put on your muscles while you train can lead to muscle growth and strength. And the stress you put on yourself to make a deadline or be on time for an appointment can make you more efficient and effective.

When daily stresses accumulate and become regular and burdensome, they can lead to anxiety, lack of motivation, irritability, depression, fatigue, headaches, muscle pain, and upset stomach. While life will never be completely stress-free, there are areas of your life that can be restructured to minimize it.

So while people often focus on reducing momentary stress, the goal should be to eliminate long-term tension—lingering thoughts, issues, and tasks that haunt you incessantly. Those stressors will ultimately do you in, healthwise.

How do you do it? You might need to make real, lasting

changes in your personal or professional life. Or you may just need to figure out how to deal with life stresses more effectively. I am a strong proponent of therapy, which can be a useful aid. Ultimately, stress reduction is a highly personal matter that requires you to be honest with yourself and take action.

I still have moments where stress gets the best of me. But I'm fortunate in that I've always found ways to power through and not allow stress to prevent me from going about my business. In fact, I believe I've always managed to appear calm even during times when I was actually boiling inside. Nowadays, I'm rarely if ever visibly upset, but when I was younger, in my 30s especially, I was more combative and prone to engaging in a heated back-and-forth during a disagreement. The entertainment business can be noisy and abusive, but as I became more personally secure, I understood that the best way to solve problems is to have gentle conversations and find commonalities, not get too stressed or react angrily. There was a time when I was calm, calm, calm, calm, calm—and then really, really, really not calm. I don't do that anymore. Along with being more aware of that side of my personality, I've also made personal choices—praying more, for example—that have helped me get rid of that boiling point.

CHAPTER 8

Find Your Killer Confidence

Looking great is the world's greatest confidence boost—period. Here's how to put your best body forward, always.

IT'S IMPOSSIBLE TO present your best self without taking pride in your appearance. Showing up to any event or activity showered, smelling good, and appropriately and neatly attired is a sign of respect for yourself and others. But don't play dress-up. Your presentation should reflect your authentic self—just not at the expense of being inappropriate in a given situation.

There are exceptions, of course. The late Apple co-founder Steve Jobs made a black mock turtleneck, blue jeans, and New

Balance sneakers his uniform for every occasion. When you're a genius like Steve Jobs, you can do those sorts of things.

And Facebook CEO Mark Zuckerberg is someone else who doesn't adhere to a traditional work attire. His penchant for hoodies and jeans helped him reduce what he called "decision fatigue," or expending energy on what he viewed as trivial decisions regarding his dress code. However, I've also seen Mark wear suits at certain events. It's not that he's selling out—he just knows how to read the room and show respect to the people he's addressing or accompanying.

Early in my career, I was more buttoned-up compared with the way I am today. Back then, I had a strict dress code for just about every business-related occasion: suit and tie. No exceptions. I was intent on dressing and portraying myself in a formal way because that's what I believed was the image of legitimacy and success. And during conversation, I would be trapped inside of my own head as my mind flipped through a Rolodex of questions: *How am I doing? Am I being admired? Do I come across as sharp and successful?*

I don't blame people if they thought I was distant or cold, but I wasn't secure enough to understand that being myself—or learning to be comfortable being myself—is a more natural way to live.

I began to move toward this mentality in my 30s. Wendy had helped me realize that it's more attractive to present yourself as you are, with your flaws and with humor. And I was working with a business coach named Gloria Henn on learning to let go of past anxieties, being more authentic, and establishing and protecting boundaries.

To this day, I still consider this area to be a work in progress, but I have worked hard to make strides. Nowadays in conversation, instead of grappling with questions about how I'm doing or how I'm being perceived, I'm more interested in how the person I'm speaking with is doing. Ultimately, gaining self-confidence and being less concerned with outside perceptions have allowed me to adopt a more casual style. I don't wear a suit and tie to the office every day. In fact, even when I make a televised media appearance, I ditch the tie. While I'm someone who believes a tie adds crispness and finishes off a look, I just don't like wearing one.

If wearing a tie makes you feel comfortable and gives you an added sense of confidence, wear a tie. Figure out how to present yourself in the best possible light—while still being comfortable and authentic. After all, a little effort goes a long way toward fostering self-confidence. As your self-confidence grows, you'll feel more assured with your appearance and body image. And positive body image has also been shown to ward off depression and unhealthy dieting behaviors.

Hop off the Scale

THE MIRROR IS a free diagnostic tool that can be used for self-assessment. In some ways it can be just as or even more important than a scale—if you like what you see, what the scale reads isn't that important. Plus, the scale's worth can diminish significantly if you use it to judge your self-worth. Remember, the scale isn't there to judge you, to make you feel bad about yourself, or to shame you into losing weight. For the best results, don't weigh yourself more than once a week, and always try to weigh yourself at the same time of day because body weight can fluctuate by three to five pounds over the course of a day.

"Positive body image has also been shown to ward off depression and unhealthy dieting behaviors."

It's also wise to keep in mind that attaining the "perfect" body isn't realistic. Focus on the things you *can* control or change, and begin with small alterations.

Use these simple ways to start feeling and looking younger without putting in too much effort.

Take the Bathing Suit Test

DO YOU FEEL comfortable in a bathing suit? If the answer is yes, you embody what a fit physique symbolizes: good health, boundless energy, confidence, and optimism. If the answer is no, revisit the answer to the question, *What do you want?*

Exercise to Erase the Years

EXERCISE CAN REJUVENATE skin. A Canadian study took skin biopsies from the buttocks* of sedentary men and women over age 65. Subjects then jogged or cycled twice a week for 30 minutes for three months. Another skin sample was taken. When the samples were compared, the post-exercise skin was now indistinguishable from the skin of 20- to 40-year-olds.

Pay Attention to Detail

I GET HAIRCUTS every three weeks, trim stray hairs when necessary, shave daily, and wear clothes that fit. Not only do I value a clean and crisp look, but it's also important in my business to look well put together. How you dress, groom, and carry yourself delivers a message to other people, so in this regard, paying attention to detail matters.

A study published in the journal *PLOS ONE* researched the impact of scent on the perception of beauty and attraction. After being shown a series of photographs that were paired with an odor, subjects rated faces associated with a pleasant smell as looking both younger and more attractive.

---

*Why the buttocks? Because the researchers wanted samples from skin that was not exposed to sunlight.

Take your spouse or partner and test fragrances that you both like. Remember that fragrances smell different on different people, so don't rely on a scent strip.

Once you find a scent you like, I recommend sticking with it. Think of it as a kind of branding. Believe it or not, you will be remembered, often unconsciously, by your scent. To this day, I remember my dad's scent (Amphora pipe tobacco) and my mom's perfume (Maja Myrurgia). If I encounter these scents now it still reminds me of them. I chose Hermès Eau d'Orange Verte before I had kids. Today, my children know my scent and associate it with me.

A BEGINNER'S GUIDE
TO HEALTH AND WELLNESS

STEP 1: Aim to consume 16 ounces of water when you get up in the morning, with meals, and before bed, adding more whenever you feel thirsty.

STEP 2: Increase your quantity and quality of sleep.

STEP 3: Take action to reduce stress.

STEP 4: Clean out your closet. Give away anything you haven't worn within the past year. Men, get your shoes polished.

WHAT'S NEXT: Work to the point where water becomes your drink of choice and you're getting seven to eight hours of sleep each night. Stay current with medical exams and take steps recommended by your doctor.

Part Four

FIND YOUR SOUL

How to discover a deeper connection with yourself and those you love

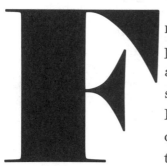**IFTEEN YEARS AGO,** I was invited to participate in the Pan-Mass Challenge, a charity bike ride in Massachusetts supporting the Dana-Farber Cancer Institute. I was new to cycling and considered myself moderately fit, but the two-day, 185-mile trek would be the most challenging physical activity I'd ever taken on. Still, I wanted to be involved and offer support after one of my cycling buddies revealed that his father was a patient at Dana-Farber before passing away from cancer at age 60.

The starting point was in Sturbridge. After a 4:30 a.m. breakfast, we rode in the dark to the starting line, where thousands of bicycles were in line waiting. I wasn't sure what to expect other than some long rides over the next 48 hours, but I received much more than that. As the ride kicked off at 6 a.m., I could see the streets were lined with supporters, many of them cancer survivors, cheering us on, holding posters and photos of loved ones who died from, survived, or were currently battling cancer. An especially touching sign read, "I survived cancer thanks to you."

This was the scene throughout all 185 miles. I had never

played competitive sports, and had really never been cheered on athletically, so it was a new experience for me. But more important, it drove home that what we were doing was truly making a difference in people's lives.

When I finished the race in Provincetown, endorphins— basically internal opiates—were running rampant in me, and I was struck by how good it felt, this intersection of challenging physical activity and human connections, and that so many of us banded together to support such a worthy cause. It was an emotional day, and I called Wendy as soon as the race finished and told her that was one of the top 20 moments of my life. Later, I found out that the Pan-Mass Challenge raises roughly $40 million each year. I knew I had to repeat it, and I did for nine more years.

The event wasn't so meaningful for me because of the route or how many calories I burned. Ultimately, the ride was defined by a spiritual experience.

In this part of the book, I'll address the three elements that I believe make up the notion of soul: human connections, spirituality, and overall energy. This discussion will not benefit from a rigid, prescribed approach and, indeed, should be deeply personal and tailored to your background and beliefs.

CHAPTER 9

Construct Your Best Support System

There's no better way to increase accountability than by surrounding yourself with an ensemble of trusted and highly motivated individuals.

IN SOME WAYS my life would be a lot easier if I went to a 6 a.m. class at my nearby Equinox. It would certainly eliminate all the organizational and administrative things I do every day to keep The Program going. But I continue to put in the work because the group has truly changed my life and body in ways I would never have achieved on my own—or even working with a personal trainer.

The experience of conquering a challenge with a tribe feels both physically and emotionally uplifting. It's more fun—even when we're all struggling. At the end of the day, I believe that at its best getting physical is a group activity, a point that is largely lost in today's culture of luxury gyms populated with people hiding behind their earbuds and Spotify accounts.

That camaraderie extends beyond the gym floor, too. To the people who make up The Program, it's more than a weekly exercise group; it's a matrix of people who count on one another in all aspects of life. We vary in age and come from various careers and athletic backgrounds, but our love of fitness keeps us connected and runs much deeper than a passion for exercise. We're a support system, and whether it's for career advice or personal advice, team members make themselves available at all times.

There is no profit motive with The Program. No money changes hands, and the group's focus is entirely on being there for one another while striving to benefit personally. So while I'm proud of my fitness accomplishments—I'm leaner, more athletic, and happier since The Program's inception—what's truly inspiring is when we see members of the group thrive: Dyan Tsiumis (page 78) shedding weight, dedicating herself to training, and taking the stage at a bikini competition; Eric Posner (page 153) and Tony Richardson (page 58) losing 15 and 20 pounds, respectively; Paul Schnell (page 84) rallying his team during one of our group fund-raising challenges.

Those are just a handful of The Program's stories that motivate me. Now, I don't want you to look at The Program and think, "Must be nice." I want you to look at The Program and think, "I want to be part of something like this."

If you were starting a business, the profit model could change, but to become successful the principles would need to remain the same. If you want a business to succeed, don't think about how you can get rich doing it; think about what that business can do that's of service to people, or how it can provide a benefit that's greater than what they pay. And then proceed to do it over and over again, better and better every day. In The Program, we invest in ourselves but devote our support to one another to help strengthen our bond and achieve our goals.

The Science of Social Connections

AS WE AGE it's common for us to lose touch with people. We have our work groups and our families, and both can be the source of incredibly valuable and meaningful relationships. I value my relationship with my wife and children above all others, as do many of us. And I have met and developed lifelong friendships with people I have worked with, as well. But it can be hard to find and maintain friends outside of these circles. I've worked hard to build nonfamily and nonwork relationships. Many of them revolve around fitness. One of my favorite adventures is an annual bike trip with friends; we ride hard and then spend our free time talking about books, politics, our personal lives, and anything else that matters to us at the moment. While the cycling is challenging and rewarding, the best part of these trips is the personal connections with people to whom I'm not related and with whom I do not work.

While some men have golf buddies or poker nights, I don't think most guys make an effort to build a group of friends or maintain the friends they have. Women are generally better at maintaining social circles, but they, too, can fall into isolation due to pressures, work obligations, and family life.

Self-Determination Theory

ACCORDING TO SELF-DETERMINATION theory, there are three components to motivation: competence, autonomy, and

Aim to better yourself and those around you.

—Eric Posner, 30, The Program

Eric had a business idea: The group cycling classes that were taking over New York City were good, but they were not capturing the opportunity to include camaraderie and competition into the fitness experience. Eric approached me and asked if he could run an idea by me—and that idea was Swerve, an indoor cycling studio that incorporates a team and competitive element. When Swerve opened, I brought some of the crew over, and we loved how Eric and Swerve approached fitness. Now Swerve is one of our regular workout destinations. We also asked Eric to join our group. A former lacrosse player at Harvard who had eaten one too many late-night pizzas, Eric quickly dropped 15 pounds and got ripped.

"Many people played team sports growing up, but when you get older, you lack that in your life," he says. "We hold each other accountable as a team and strive to get better together. I quickly realized that this group was more than just a bunch of people who wake up early to work out together, but a crew of mindful athletes looking to better themselves and those around them. When we attend classes, the energy of the room is high and contagious. Outside of class, we're pretty active on social media, posting about our workouts, our progress, or group photos because we know the impact it has on others."

relatedness. Competence implies that it's important to be able to have some success at the task at hand. Autonomy means having a measure of control over the decisions you're making. If your boss is a micromanager and you have no ability to make decisions, take risks, or try new things, you likely won't stay motivated for long, no matter how competent you are.

The third factor of motivational theory is relatedness—being connected to other people. A sense of community. A "we're in it together" feeling that helps power you through obstacles and tough challenges. When all three factors work together, you experience what experts call intrinsic motivation, which comes from within, as opposed to extrinsic motivation, which is tied to goals established with or by others.

Relatedness doesn't just help motivate you—it's an asset to well-being. Researchers from the University of North Carolina found that the more social ties people had at an early age, the better their health was at the beginning and the end of their lives. And the size of a person's social network was shown to influence health in early and late adulthood. In adolescence, social isolation increased the risk of inflammation by the same amount as physical inactivity, while social integration protected against abdominal obesity. In the elderly, social isolation was shown to be more harmful to health than diabetes. In middle age, it wasn't the number of social connections that mattered, but rather what those connections provided in terms of social support.

"A tribe changes your body, improves your health, and enriches your soul."

Another study, which was published in the journal *Psychology and Aging*, found that the *quantity* of social interactions a person has at age 20—and the *quality* of social relationships that person has at age 30—can both benefit his or her well-being later in life.

Data supports the notion that strong social networks have a lasting impact on health. A meta-analytic review conducted by researchers from Brigham Young University analyzed more than 148 studies to determine that stronger social relationships increased survival rates by 50 percent. Having fewer friends or weak social ties to the community was shown to be just as harmful to health as being an alcoholic, smoking nearly a pack of cigarettes a day, failing to exercise, or suffering from obesity.

Enhance Relatedness by Creating a Tribe

I LOVE WHAT The Program represents. I look forward to my daily workouts as well as social interactions with team members. I can't tell you exactly where everyone in our crew will be in 10 or 20 years, but I'm willing to bet that many of us will still be in touch, still be training together, and still be part of this amazing web of relationships. You don't have to have The Program, but consider having something.

To make and sustain smart choices, and to combine them into an ageless lifestyle, you need social support. The right mix of people gives you three things you can't get on your own:

1) **Accountability**

   Do you have a plan to wake up early to work out? Sounds easy until the alarm sounds and it's still dark out. A social network consisting of people who have committed to meet at 6 a.m. trumps going back to sleep. This is the most commonly appreciated benefit of The Program. We hold one another accountable, not in a judgmental way, but in a way that makes you want to do well—because you want to show up for your team. This is a foundation for lasting motivation.

2) **Support**

   When things aren't going well or as planned, it's easy to bury your sorrows in a beer or a dish of ice cream. Unfortunately, that solace is usually fleeting. But what happens when somebody talks you through whatever issue you're having, perhaps offering advice, an encouraging word, or just listening and giving you a hug? This can be a lot more comforting, helpful, and long-lasting. Knowing you don't have to handle your struggles alone is half the battle to overcoming them.

3) Motivation

In The Program, no one is ever unpleasant to anyone else. No unkind words are spoken. While we can be warmly competitive, there is no mean-spirited trash-talking. Negativity just isn't tolerated. If you can't handle that, you don't fit in. But, there is a difference between negativity and a nudge. Sometimes you need a push to get through a tough workout. Sometimes you need a reminder that getting hammered every Friday night will derail your goals. Sometimes you need to be encouraged to try a little harder at work.

A tribe can take different forms. The Program is currently a group of about 80, with maybe 15 to 20 people attending each workout. Occasionally, the larger group will get together socially for events like dinners, volunteering efforts, and charity fundraisers. This is one of many ways to structure a tribe. If you don't currently have a tribe, consider developing one or joining an existing one. For sustained motivation, make sure it's an activity you enjoy. The activity doesn't have to be exercise-based, but I think that can be especially valuable. And if it transitions into something deeper than training, that's great, and, over time, that's the way it should work. Some possibilities:

◆ **Recruit a training partner**
Ask a reliable buddy who has similar goals, abilities, and availability in his or her schedule to exercise regularly—

Always strive to get to the next level.

—Nick Sizer, 28, The Program

Six years ago, Nick graduated from Connecticut College, where he had played lacrosse and water polo, and moved to New York City ready to attack his new career. Nick and I met at Flywheel, an indoor cycling studio.

"I remember thinking: How could a 50-something man be *this* fit?" Nick says. "And why did he look like Bruce Wayne after lifting?"

Spin class with Nick eventually grew into the scheduled workouts that now form the foundation of The Program, and that evolved into much more than a fitness group, but rather a community in which fitness and life goals meet. Nick was one of the first people who truly understood that I got as much out of the group as everyone else did—in that it kept me hungry, fresh with ideas, and passionate. Nick has served as one of our main leaders—pushing, laughing, and helping others pursue their goals while he pursues his.

"We now sit six years after this little experiment kicked off, currently with about 80 people on our roster. Some old, some young, some short, some tall, some coordinated, some not. One thing has always remained constant: Everyone is working to get to the next level," he says. "It's our new team. It's given me consistency, some incredible role models, some lifelong friends, and a crew I can always count on. I'm thankful every day for the role and influence it plays in my life and hope that I can give back 1 percent of what it gives me."

lift weights, shoot hoops, or engage in another activity that piques both of your interests.

◆ **Start a fitness group**
Any activity that gets a group together—doubles tennis, mountain biking, a lunchtime running group—will increase the odds that you'll keep showing up. A potential downside: Competition can sometimes take over. Be sure to choose people who can compete hard but with maturity and kindness.

◆ **Join an existing fitness group**
If you'd rather find a larger fitness or sports group than create and organize your own, Meetup (meetup.com), Eventbrite (eventbrite.com), OurPlan (ourplanapp.com), and Wiith (wiithapp.com) can help. Local gyms, YMCAs, and adventure clubs are also worth exploring. Or you can ask friends who are fit where they train and with whom they work out.

You'll notice I did not suggest significant other or spouse as one of the possible social groups. While I don't think you should exclude your romantic partner from your health goals, it can be a dangerous area for some couples. First, a romantic partnership has so many variables that throwing in athletic goals only adds to those complexities. When a spouse needs a hug but you give her a nudge, the interaction isn't perceived the same way as it would be if it were with a friend. There's too much background noise that can influence these interactions.

Second, and this is more important, men need to be better about developing and keeping social connections outside of family and work. So having a tribe with a shared mission of optimum health and fitness can be a life changer.

A tribe changes your body, improves your health, and enriches your soul.

CHAPTER

10

Embrace Your Spiritual Side

Whatever you believe, becoming
a calmer, more patient, and more tolerant
person is a huge step toward not only
self-fulfillment, but also great health.

INSECURITY, FAILURE, WORRY about the future and how things will turn out—yes, I experience all those things. I'm assuming you do as well. But I have reached a point where those feelings of discontent are not debilitating or overpowering. Finding this inner peace wasn't connected to a business or financial success, either. Adding spirituality to my life over the past decade has helped me make a conscious effort to recognize and remind myself that things may not turn out the way I expect or want them to. And when that happens, I'll still be OK.

I don't believe in big epiphanies or spectacular instances of change. Usually, we look back at what we perceive as enlightening moments and realize they weren't as impactful as we had hoped. So there wasn't one specific event that I credit with my becoming more spiritual but, more accurately, an accumulation of advice from close friends, having an open mind, and the trajectory my life took after I decided to live more healthfully. I don't take the position of "I'm old and experienced and successful, so I've got it all figured out." I feel as though I can—and do—learn something from anyone I meet. In business, mentors of mine include Don Gogel, who's in the private equity business, Barry Diller, who's in the digital media business, and Dick Parsons, who was the CEO of Time Warner. These three people have had a great impact on me professionally. That's not to say they haven't taught me things personally, but, in my personal life, it's friends, friends of friends, family, my workout buddies—if I have a relationship with someone, chances are high I've been fortunate enough to learn something from them. In that way, I feel mentored.

Over the past decade, I've made a larger effort to remind myself to open not just my mind but also my heart and soul to relationships with people of all different sorts, of all different ages, with all different careers. Doing so has allowed me to become more humble, relaxed, and understanding, as I truly feel like I have learned and continue to learn from everyone.

The addition of morning prayer has added more depth to my spirituality. Before I move forward, I do want to address that I understand spirituality is more personal than deciding the foods to eliminate or arranging a cheat meal schedule. What you believe (or choose not to believe) and what you practice are generally based on your background, education, and upbringing. I'd be an unlikely proselyte on a good day. I don't have the background or credentials, never mind the inclination, to try to sell you on religion. I'm Jewish by background, and I feel connected to that religion and am happy to describe myself that way, but my daily practice of silent prayer is a spiritual practice, not a religious practice. I didn't start doing it because I thought or hoped someone else was listening to me, but I continued doing it once I realized it had helped me in a way that nothing else did.

At age 55, I longed for a deeper connection with the world. Inspired by introspective discussions with friends, I began dedicating a few minutes every morning to silent prayer, when I'd reflect on what's important and think about my life and the greater world. I find that my morning ritual grounds me in a way that nothing else does.

Though I feel I've always been a reasonably calm, patient, and tolerant guy, many people noticed that I became even more so after I integrated quiet morning prayer into my life. When I reach a tipping point of frustration, I no longer raise my voice or argue angrily. And rather than judge someone who's different from me or who just doesn't appeal to me, I try to have empathy and look beyond outward appearances to consider reasons that that person may act the way he or she does. These days, morning prayer helps me center myself and focus on my goals and actions—but not the things I can't control—and therefore has vastly decreased my stress levels and increased my overall happiness.

> **"I believe everyone should include some form of quiet reflection in his or her life."**

I can't guarantee you'll experience the same outcome, but it wouldn't surprise me. And that's the reason why I believe everyone should include some form of quiet reflection in his or her life. Reflection during which you relax, let go, think about where you fit into this world, and consider how you're influencing the greater good. This book has so far been about taking action: Eat this, stay away from that, sleep more, sweat, get regular checkups. When you do, you will see results. The implication is that you control the outcomes. However, I deeply believe that's only half the story. You also have to acknowledge that some things occur no matter what you do or what choices you make. It's the way life works. So my definition of spirituality is to understand that there are bigger forces at play that are well outside your control.

This approach makes you more mindful of the people around you. It makes you a better listener and decision maker and may even help you become wiser. Certainly, it helps you put life into perspective so you can balance your work obligations with what's really important—your family and your relationships. And so it helps reduce stress and allows you to live a healthier life.

The big reason to engage in some kind of quiet reflection is to release your mind and feel the things that are greater than you are as an individual. And there's plenty of evidence that this kind of spiritual practice has great benefits:

Spirituality Reduces Anxiety

RESEARCHERS FROM THE University of São Paulo in Brazil sought to investigate the effects of prayer on health. Several specific beneficial effects were identified, including reducing the anxiety of mothers with cancer-stricken children. Another study concluded that what you expect from prayer might influence its effect. Researchers at Baylor University analyzed data from 1,714 individuals. The study focused on general anxiety, social anxiety, obsession, and compulsion. Those who prayed to a loving and supportive God who they thought would be there to comfort and protect them were less likely to show symptoms of anxiety-related disorders than those who prayed but did not expect God to comfort or protect them.

Spirituality Improves Health

A **STUDY BY** researchers from Massachusetts General Hospital and published in the journal *PLOS ONE* found that individuals in relaxation-response-focused training programs that included yoga, meditation, and prayer used an average of 43 percent fewer health care services in the year after their participation than in the preceding year. Another study from Northern Arizona University backs up those findings: Researchers examined the relationship between meditation and psychological mindfulness and physical health in 177 adults with Buddhist experience and determined that meditating on a regular basis and having a greater experience with Buddhism was related to higher psychological mindfulness scores. Researchers also found that meditating strengthened immunity and reduced depression. The findings were published in the *Journal of Happiness Studies*.

Spirituality Improves Memory

A **STUDY PUBLISHED** in the journal *Psychiatry Research* found that an eight-week mindfulness meditation program appeared to yield measurable changes in brain regions associated with memory, sense of self, empathy, and stress. In the small study, MRIs found increased gray matter density in the hippocampus, which is important for learning and memory, and in structures associated with self-awareness, compassion, and introspection. Participants also reported reductions in stress.

You can and should approach spirituality in any way you like; there are numerous ways to add it to your life:

Find strength in numbers.

—Erica Schultz, 39, The Program

E rica was hired to photograph one of The Program's workouts for a feature in *Muscle & Fitness* magazine. She knew next to nothing about The Program, except that "it was a crew made up of extremely attractive, fit, and motivated people who liked to train all over the city at the crazy hour of 6 a.m." Her job was to capture as many images as possible, and the hustle she displayed to keep up with the fast-paced workout left her exhausted and dripping with sweat. But she was also inspired by the energy and intensity of the group. It wasn't long before Erica and her husband, Zack Zeigler (page 46)— the writer of the *M&F* piece—became regulars. "I'm much stronger than I was before I started training with The Program, and I'm able to push myself harder than I ever thought," she says. "These people are my fitness family."

- **Group prayer and worship**
  Traditional services and formal approaches to religion.

- **Individualized prayer**
  Reflecting quietly by yourself.

- **Meditation**
  Sit comfortably in a chair or cross-legged on the floor. Shut your eyes and bring your attention to your breath coming in and going out. If you get distracted—and you will—simply begin again.

- **Deep breathing**
  In a relaxing pose or lying down, focus on deep inhalation and exhalation. Try to clear your mind.

- **Yoga**
  Many people practice yoga—combining breathing and stretching techniques and poses—not only for its physical benefits, but also for its spiritual component.

Whichever method you choose, go in with an open mind. Take three to five minutes every morning or evening when you're alone. Try it for a few weeks and see how it feels. My guess is you will decide that it really makes a difference.

CHAPTER 11

Harness Your Good Energy

Make sure you always have enough gas in the tank to work hard, excel, get ahead, be strong, and stay focused every day.

I **MAY BE TIRED** when I wake up around 5 a.m. to train with The Program, but I'm prepared both mentally and physically to push through inertia. There is no question that the reason I feel that way is because of the way I live—I consume the right foods, generally get enough rest, and manage my stress levels. I treat my body, mind, and soul with respect, and I avoid toxic substances and behaviors. As a result, I can usually run all day—efficiently, effectively, happily.

This is what I mean by being better, faster, stronger, and ageless. It's about possessing vitality, minimizing disease risk, and maintaining an attractive body that looks and feels the same way—or even better than—it did decades ago.

It all comes down to energy. Do you have enough to work hard and excel? To operate with passion? To serve others? To be motivated and motivating? To meet obligations? To be happy? Do you have enough energy to live the way you want to live? When you do, the strategies I've outlined become self-reinforcing.

If you're hurting yourself—eating too much junk, not exercising enough, staying up too late, drinking too much booze—it can be hard to get started. This is why I suggest being gentle with yourself and easing into change. Even one small step is forward movement. Once you exchange inertia for momentum, once you start doing everything better, from eating to sweating, the motion accelerates. Energy builds and builds upon itself, so it doesn't take as much effort to sustain maximum speed.

Research confirms that energy, broadly defined, matters. A study published in the journal *Population Health Management* found that employees who consumed unhealthy diets, smoked, and exercised less were much less productive compared with their colleagues with healthier habits.

And that's just about *workplace* productivity; that's not even considering the energy drain that influences other areas of your life, such as social networks and romantic relationships, in which the barometer isn't really productivity but rather satisfaction.

What we're after is using major lifestyle decisions and actions to create the energy you want in life. And if you follow these suggestions you are highly likely to succeed. That said, there are a number of additional tactics you can employ to practice good energy hygiene and improve performance. Here are a few:

◆ **Keep a tidy workspace**

I try to be thoughtful about the way guests and visitors feel upon arrival in my office by keeping my workplace neat, clean, and smelling good. If you go to the bathroom at ZMC, it's clean. I get annoyed when it's not—it may be the only time people can see me visibly frustrated. It's that important to me because I want guests to know how much their comfort means. No matter what resources you have available or the type of work environment you're in, keeping a tidy, organized workplace will reduce anxiety and stress.

Consider adding plants to a room or an office, too. According to a study published in the journal *Environmental Health Perspectives*, people who work in well-ventilated offices with below-average levels of indoor pollutants and carbon dioxide (CO_2) have significantly higher cognitive functioning scores—in crucial areas such as responding to a crisis or developing strategy—than those who work in offices with typical levels. They found that cognitive performance scores for participants who worked in the greener environments were, on average, double those of participants who worked in the conventional settings.

◆ **Nap as needed**

Once all three kids left home for college I was able to add naps into my weekend schedule. It's not a regular thing, but when I nap for about an hour, I feel refreshed. I know research suggests that 10 to 20 minutes is the ideal time to nap for increased energy, and that going for too long or drifting into deep sleep will make you groggy and sluggish. But an hour seems to be my magic number. During the workday, an hour isn't as realistic, so if your work environment allows for naps, cap it at 20 minutes to get a late-day energy boost.

Take pride in your accomplishments.

—*Christie Posner, 32, The Program*

A few years ago on Christmas, Christie worked out with her brother, Eric Posner (page 153). It was the most challenging workout she'd ever completed. Afterward, the two shared a photo on Facebook. Although he was looking jacked, her arms became the topic of conversation. The number of positive comments she received awakened something deep inside her—a desire to achieve even more success.

Christie was competitive growing up, but when she was 14, she tore her ACL and meniscus playing basketball. After nine months of rehab, she tore the same ACL and meniscus in preseason lacrosse.

"In relation to sports, I was never the same, mentally," she says. "I convinced myself that being able to dance all night in high heels was somehow a less-dangerous risk, which sadly enabled me to give up on team sports completely."

Now with The Program, she loves being part of a team again.

"I truly learned the importance of how much 'I am proud of you' really means," she says. "Living a life of focus, determination, goal setting, support, and fun has made me a better person. Each day I get better and better, and it is a mission of mine to bring anyone along with me."

- ◆ **Get up and go**

    Sitting for too long is not good for you. Besides being tough on your back, it's associated with inactivity and adverse health effects. Using a stand-up desk is one option, but they can be pricey. So if purchasing one isn't feasible, make it a goal to get up and walk around at least once every 45 to 60 minutes. Focusing on something for an hour or so, you'll most likely benefit from a break to maintain a desired level of productivity. If you find that productivity is lagging, you are much better served taking a break and walking than trying to power through.

Some Final Thoughts on Energy

NOW YOU KNOW where I stand when it comes to all the components that serve as my main principles for living healthy and strong. That's not the main point of this book, to implore you to work out a dozen times a week or to eat everything I eat, though it might not hurt to try. The point is for you to take these principles and find ways to apply them to your life, to grow, to get better, to use the good that you're developing and turn it into an incredibly satisfying life.

Perhaps the most important thing for you to think about is what kind of life you want and what will make you happy. If food, exercise, and sleep are the main building blocks of sustained energy, then there's one thing that serves as the ultimate power booster: setting consistent, frequent, and even hard-to-reach goals. Complacency is the enemy of fulfillment.

If you ask everyone in The Program what the most valuable part of our group is, not one of them would say it's the burpees. They—men and women, young and old—would universally agree that establishing and trying hard to achieve training, career, and life goals is the most valuable part. The quest—through workouts, a supportive community, mentoring, coaching, and discipline—drives our energy every day. It's what gets people out of bed at 5 a.m. to do brutal workouts. It's what makes people love to help one another. It's what stimulates motivation and inspiration to do something positive when taking the easy way out would be tempting. Life changes when you get your mind right. When you get your mind right, you get your body right. When you get your body right, you get your energy right. And when you put them all together, that's when you've figured out that *Becoming Ageless* isn't about redefining your age. It's about living your very best life and fulfilling your potential.

So whatever stage you're in or whatever shape you're in, the first thing you must do for sustained energy is figure out what you want and then map out your journey to get there.

I would suggest that you have multiple levels of goals— some big, some small, some with long time frames, and some with short ones. The worst thing that we can do is stop moving ahead, and, too often, that's what a lot of us do. We go through the motions as we try to keep up with work, bills, and responsibilities. But if you are specific, set yourself up for success, and are gentle with yourself as you embark on a new journey, in 90 days you can and will see major, lasting changes that allow you to feel better, recover faster, and, ultimately, live a stronger life.

After you reach 90 days, your habits will have solidified and you will be on your way toward presenting your best self and living a healthy and energized lifestyle.

A BEGINNER'S GUIDE
TO FINDING YOUR SOUL

STEP 1:   Spend 2 to 3 minutes three mornings a week committed to quiet reflection or prayer.

STEP 2:   Call a like-minded friend and schedule a workout that you'll do together. It doesn't matter if it's walking, taking a bike ride, or hitting tennis balls—just do something active.

STEP 3:   Increase your quiet meditation to 5 days a week.

STEP 4:   Come up with a strategy to include one group workout a week, whether it's with one friend or a small group.

WHAT'S NEXT: Engage in quiet meditation for 3 minutes every day and train with friends or a group 1 or 2 days a week. You'll feel much better about yourself—and the world around you.

THE ROAD AHEAD: A DIARY ENTRY FROM APRIL 7, 2017

Eighteen members of The Program took part in today's 45-minute total-body, partner circuit workout. I was catching my breath during a one-minute break and thinking about my exercise form. I've told you before that I'm my harshest critic, but I had nothing to criticize: During the previous round of exercises, every one, start to finish, rep after rep, I gave it my all and used strict and proper form—something I would have never been able to accomplish five years ago. And then I thought about my workout session the day before, when a trainer challenged me to complete 100 push-ups in five minutes. I finished in four.

Now, for teenagers or people who consider themselves athletes, that type of progress wouldn't be surprising. But I'm 60 years old and have never considered myself an athlete. Yet these movements have become second nature, and I am continuing to get fitter. Someone's typical reaction to learning this? "That's impossible! You're not supposed to gain any skills at 60—your skills are supposed to be declining."

It's simply not true, and it serves as another reminder that age should not define how competent you can be.

As the workout resumed I remained tuned into my efforts, but I paid attention to what was going on around me: Seeing the team exchange high-fives and pass out fist bumps and hearing them encourage one another to finish strong were both moving and inspiring. Afterward, we took a team picture, and—this is going to be tough to explain without sounding like I'm proselytizing or being phony—as we broke for the day my takeaway wasn't, *Wow, that was an amazing workout.* It was, *Wow, that was an amazing way to start my day—with an incredible group of positive and wonderful people who are all leaving in high spirits to do the best they can in the world.*

I know that sounds corny, but I truly believe people leave our group saying, *How can I have a really good day? How can I spread goodwill? How can I be of service to others?*

I may be projecting, but that's how I feel, and I feel as though making small but numerous positive changes in your lifestyle in order to live a healthier and fitter life certainly has the ability to leave you with a similar feeling of satisfaction. As you move forward, through your ups and downs of recalibrating your life, I'd like you to remember something: Anything is possible, except perfection. If you're willing to take a chance on believing that notion and dedicate yourself to experimenting with a new approach to life without judging yourself, I believe you'll be amazed at the result.

You don't need to follow my intense fitness regimen, eat the same foods I eat, or mimic what we do in The Program to experience substantial change, either. You don't need to get the living hell kicked out of you at early-morning boot camps, or limp out of a class bruised and battered, to be productive. But when good people surround you, and you're gentle with yourself and accept that it's OK to aspire to be the best and fall short so long as you pick yourself up and try again the next day—that seems like a great metaphor for life.

Part Five

BECOME AGELESS

Strategies for eating and working out that support health, longevity, and your goal of a leaner and more muscular body

The Becoming Ageless Eating Plan

Learn to develop better eating habits and discover healthy and delicious recipes to prepare for any meal—even dessert.

A LTHOUGH **66 DAYS** is the average time for making a new behavior automatic, it often takes between 18 and 254 days, according to research from the University College London. If you're unable to adopt a new dietary guideline, ease into it month by month. Here's how:

- **Decide the target body weight you wish to reach**
  Figure out your caloric needs by multiplying your goal weight by 12. (So a person aiming to weigh 180 pounds should plan to consume around 2,160 calories each day.) Look to reach that caloric goal by the second week of your reboot.

- **Eat three meals per day**
  Use the unlimited and limited categories from page 94 with a focus on consuming more fibrous and protein-centric foods. If it takes a week or two to adjust to three meals, that's fine. Eliminate breaded, deep-fried, and processed foods or reserve them for cheat days.

- **Drink more water**
  Drink a large glass of water about 15 to 30 minutes before you eat and then two more glasses during your meal. Overall, try to consume at least 16 more ounces of water per day than you did before your reboot period began. Refrain from drinking soda and sugary juices on non-cheat days.

- **Experiment with a cheat schedule**
  Finding the one that works best for you might take a few weeks. (See suggestions on page 122.)

If you want more structure, use the seven-day eating plan on the next page as a guideline. A month in, you should be in full swing and, hopefully, staying the course.

The *Becoming Ageless* 7-Day Eating Plan

Meal	Monday	Tuesday	Wednesday
Breakfast	■ 2 eggs (poached or hard/soft-boiled) ■ Bowl of berries ■ Small cup of low-fat cottage cheese or nonfat plain yogurt	■ 2 eggs (poached or hard/soft-boiled) ■ Apple slices ■ Small cup of low-fat cottage cheese or nonfat plain yogurt	■ 3 strips of bacon or 4 ounces of grilled chicken breast ■ Orange segments ■ Small cup of low-fat cottage cheese or nonfat plain yogurt
Lunch	■ Large salad with vegetables (no cheese or croutons) and lemon juice and vinegar ■ 6 ounces of grilled chicken ■ Steamed broccoli	■ 6 ounces of poached or grilled salmon ■ Steamed vegetables ■ Rice	■ Large salad with vegetables (no cheese or croutons) and lemon juice and vinegar ■ 6 ounces of grilled chicken
Optional Snack	■ 20 almonds	■ Bowl of berries	■ Apple slices with PB2 peanut butter ■ Low-fat cottage cheese
Dinner	■ 6 ounces of grilled fish ■ Steamed vegetables ■ Rice	■ 6 ounces of roasted or grilled pork loin ■ Grilled vegetables ■ 1 small roasted yam	■ 6 ounces of poached or grilled fish ■ Steamed vegetables ■ 1 small roasted yam

178

Thursday	Friday	Saturday	Sunday
■ Nonfat plain yogurt with fresh berries ■ 2 eggs (poached or hard/ soft-boiled)	■ Smoothie (see pages 204– 205 for recipes) ■ Small cup of low-fat cottage cheese or nonfat plain yogurt	■ 2 eggs (poached or hard/soft-boiled), apple slices with PB2 peanut butter ■ Small cup of low-fat cottage cheese or nonfat plain yogurt ■ 3 strips of bacon	■ Cheat with a small portion of pancakes or French toast using minimal butter and syrup ■ 3 strips of bacon
FAST-FOOD OPTION: ■ Grilled chicken sandwich (no bun) ■ Side salad (ask for it with no cheese) with dressing on the side	■ Cheat with 1 slice of pizza (as many vege-table toppings as you like) ■ Large salad with vegetables (no cheese or croutons) and lemon juice and vinegar	**RESTAURANT OPTION:** ■ Hamburger (no bun) ■ Side of steamed vegetables (ask for it to be cooked without butter)	■ Large salad with vegetables (no cheese or croutons) and lemon juice and vinegar
■ 20 almonds ■ Nonfat plain yogurt	■ Apple slices with PB2 peanut butter	■ Bowl of berries	■ 1 ounce of cheddar cheese with small portion of plain nonfat yogurt
■ 3-egg omelet with vegetables and a small amount of cheese ■ 3 strips of bacon	■ 6 ounces of poached or grilled salmon ■ Steamed vegetables ■ 1 small roasted yam ■ Large salad with vegetables (no cheese or croutons) and lemon juice and vinegar	■ 6 ounces of lean grilled or roasted meat ■ Steamed vegetables ■ Rice ■ Large salad with vegetables (no cheese or croutons) and lemon juice and vinegar	■ 6 ounces of grilled chicken ■ Steamed vegetables ■ 1 small roasted yam

PAIR THESE FOODS TO STIFLE HUNGER

Smart snacking involves thought and preparation. Unless you have a good cafeteria at work that stays open past 3 p.m., you'll have to bring your snacks with you. The key is to plan ahead. For snacks that will keep hunger away for hours, combine something full of slow-absorbing carbohydrates with something rich in protein and with a little fat.

Here are some suggestions. Mix and match from the following columns:

CARBS	PROTEIN/FAT
1 cup celery sticks	1 Tbsp reduced-fat cream cheese spread
4 dates	7 almonds
4 whole-wheat crackers	Whey protein drink
5 strawberries	1 cup low-fat yogurt
1 cup raw baby carrots	2 Tbsp hummus
1 medium apple	1 Tbsp peanut butter
¼ cup trail mix	1 cup 1% or low-fat chocolate milk
1 whole-wheat tortilla	2 slices turkey breast and 1 slice Swiss cheese
1 pear	1 stick low-fat string cheese
1 cup berries	1-oz square hard cheese

The Becoming Ageless
RECIPES

USUALLY, IT'S WHEN we're stumped for what to eat that we fall into the trap of relying on takeout or quick heat-and-serve processed foods. That's why having a well of go-to recipes that you can rely on to provide muscle-building protein, satisfying fats, and blood-sugar-stabilizing fiber makes eating healthy easier. Keep your nutrition goals on target and your belly in check by working healthy recipes like these into your weekly meal plan:

Hard-Boiled Eggs
With Apple Slices and Cottage Cheese

INGREDIENTS

2	eggs
1	Granny Smith apple, sliced
2 Tbsp	PB2 mixed with water
6 oz	low-fat cottage cheese

DIRECTIONS

Fill a large saucepan with water and bring to a boil over medium-high heat.

Carefully lower eggs into water using a spoon and let them cook for 10 minutes.

Remove eggs from hot water and run them under cold water.

Eat eggs with apple slices spread with PB2 and round out meal with cottage cheese.

Makes 1 serving

Greek Yogurt
With Hard-Boiled Eggs and Fresh Fruit

INGREDIENTS

1 cup	nonfat plain Greek yogurt or 6 oz low-fat cottage cheese
2	hard-boiled eggs
½ cup	blueberries
½	grapefruit

DIRECTIONS

Consume individually or mix fruit with Greek yogurt.

Makes 1 serving

Egg-White Frittata

INGREDIENTS

1 Tbsp	olive oil
1 medium	onion, chopped
4 cups	chopped mixed vegetables (broccoli, carrots, cauliflower, asparagus, or your choice of other vegetables), steamed
12	egg whites
2 Tbsp	grated Parmesan cheese
1–2 cups	chopped arugula

DIRECTIONS

Preheat oven to 350°F.

Heat olive oil in a cast-iron skillet or cast-iron saucepan over medium heat.

Add onions and sauté until translucent.

Add vegetables, pour egg whites over, and cook over medium heat for 2 minutes.

Remove from heat and sprinkle Parmesan cheese on frittata.

Place frittata in oven and bake for 30 minutes, or until slightly brown on top.

Remove from oven, sprinkle chopped arugula on top of the frittata, and serve.

Makes 6 servings

Tuna Salad

INGREDIENTS

1 can	chunk light tuna packed in water, drained
1 Tbsp	fresh lemon juice
1 Tbsp	low-fat mayonnaise
	Salt and pepper, to taste

DIRECTIONS

Mix together all ingredients in a bowl.

Makes 1 serving

Roasted Turkey Wrap

INGREDIENTS

¼ lb	roasted skinless turkey breast, sliced
1–2	Boston lettuce leaves
	Mustard, to taste

DIRECTIONS

Place sliced roasted turkey breast inside of lettuce leaf, add mustard, and roll up. If desired, roll in another lettuce leaf.

Makes 1 serving

Lean Chili

INGREDIENTS

1 Tbsp	olive oil
1 large	onion, chopped
1 Tbsp	chopped garlic
¾ cup	finely chopped carrots
1 lb	bison or extra-lean beef, chopped
1 lb	lean turkey, chopped
¼ tsp	cayenne pepper
2 Tbsp	chili powder
2 tsp	ground cumin
	Salt, pepper, and crushed red pepper, to taste
1	28-oz can diced tomatoes
1	6-oz can tomato puree
1	15½-oz can kidney beans, drained

Heat olive oil in a soup pot over medium heat. Add onion and garlic and sauté until onions are translucent.

Add carrots and sauté until softened.

Add bison and lean turkey and sauté for about 7 minutes, or until cooked through.

Add remaining ingredients, stir well, and bring to a boil.

Reduce heat to simmer and cover for 30 to 60 minutes. Serve, or refrigerate for up to one week; freeze if not planning to consume dish for weeks or longer.

Makes 6–8 servings

Eggplant Parmesan

INGREDIENTS

2	whole eggplants, peeled
	Canola oil, as needed
2	8-oz packs low-fat shredded mozzarella cheese
1	32-oz jar tomato sauce (look for a prepared sauce, preferably organic with no sugar added and the lowest fat content)
¾ cup	grated Parmesan cheese
	Salt and crushed red pepper, to taste

Preheat oven to 350°F. Slice eggplant into 1-inch rounds.

Heat a cast-iron skillet over medium-high heat until smoking. Working in batches, sauté slices in a small amount of canola oil until browned on both sides.

Remove and set aside.

When you've sautéed all the eggplant slices, layer into a glass baking dish in this order: eggplant slices, mozzarella cheese, tomato sauce, grated Parmesan, and spices.

Place dish in oven and bake for 40 minutes, or until hot throughout.

Makes 4 servings

Roast Chicken

INGREDIENTS

Pinch of salt and pepper

1 lb   whole chicken

DIRECTIONS

Put a cast-iron skillet in oven and heat at 500°F for 15 minutes.

Sprinkle salt and pepper on chicken, then add to skillet. (Make sure anything the butcher left in the cavity has been removed and that the chicken has been washed and patted dry.)

Place chicken in oven and roast for 55 minutes. Remove from oven and let cool in skillet for 10 minutes before transferring to a platter.

Makes 3–4 servings

Grilled Steak

INGREDIENTS

1 tsp	canola oil
6 oz	grilled steak
1 cup	steamed vegetables
1 medium	yam

DIRECTIONS

Heat a cast-iron skillet over medium-high heat until smoking.

Add canola oil.

Add steak and cook for 2 to 3 minutes per side, or until brown. Remove, then transfer to a platter.

Cover with aluminum foil for 5 minutes, then serve.

Serve with a Roasted Yam (page 197) and Steamed Vegetables (page 198), if desired.

Makes 1 serving

Baked Salmon

INGREDIENTS

6 oz	salmon
½ Tbsp	olive oil
	Salt and pepper, to taste

DIRECTIONS

Preheat oven to 350°F.

Cover a baking sheet with aluminum foil or parchment paper.

Place salmon skin-side down on baking sheet.

Rub with olive oil.

Sprinkle with salt and pepper.

Bake for 13 minutes, then serve.

Makes 1 serving

Sautéed Zucchini

INGREDIENTS

1 Tbsp	canola oil
1 large	zucchini, thinly sliced
	Fresh lemon juice, to taste
	Soy sauce, to taste
	Salt and pepper, to taste

DIRECTIONS

Heat canola oil in a cast-iron skillet over medium heat.

Add zucchini slices and sauté until browned and softened.

Add lemon juice, soy sauce, salt, and pepper, to taste.

Stir until combined, then serve.

Makes 1 serving

White Rice

INGREDIENTS

1 cup	water
1 tsp	salt
½ cup	white long-grain rice (not "converted")

DIRECTIONS

Bring water to a boil in a small saucepan over high heat.

Add salt.

Stir in rice.

Bring to a boil again (will happen almost immediately).

Reduce heat to lowest simmer and cover.

Cook for 20 minutes.

Remove from heat. Fluff rice with fork. Cover again and let sit for 5 minutes.

Makes 1 serving

Roasted Yam

INGREDIENTS

1 large   yam

DIRECTIONS

Preheat oven to 425°F.

Wash yam with cold water and prick a few times with a fork.

Place yam on aluminum foil on oven rack.

Roast for 90 minutes.

Makes 1 serving

Steamed Vegetables

INGREDIENTS

Choose any vegetable and use any quantity (within reason)

Fresh lemon juice, to taste

Salt and pepper, to taste

DIRECTIONS

Add 2 to 3 inches of water to a pot and place a Chinese steamer over pot.

Bring water to a boil over high heat, then set to simmer.

Add vegetables, cover, and cook for 3 to 4 minutes, or until vegetables are softened.

Transfer vegetables to a bowl. Sprinkle on lemon juice, salt, and pepper.

Makes 1 serving

Side Salad

INGREDIENTS

Choose any lettuce and vegetable and use any quantity (within reason)

Salt and pepper, to taste

1 Tbsp   fresh lemon juice

1 Tbsp   red wine vinegar

DIRECTIONS

Put lettuce and vegetables in a bowl.

Add salt and pepper to taste.

Toss salad with lemon juice and red wine vinegar or make one of the healthy dressings listed on pages 202–203.

Makes 1 serving

Grilled Chicken Salad

INGREDIENTS

	Choose any lettuce and vegetable and use any quantity (within reason)
4 oz	grilled chicken, chopped
1 Tbsp	fresh lemon juice
1 Tbsp	red wine vinegar

DIRECTIONS

Put lettuce, vegetables, and grilled chicken in a bowl.

Toss salad with lemon juice and red wine vinegar, or make either of the healthy dressings listed in this book on pages 202–203.

Makes 1 serving

Vegetable Salad

INGREDIENTS

2 cups	arugula
1 tsp	fresh dill
3 5	cherry tomatoes
1	scallion, sliced
¼	cucumber, sliced
1	celery stalk, sliced
	Pinch of crumbled feta cheese

DIRECTIONS

Chop all ingredients except feta cheese.

Put into a bowl, add feta cheese, and toss. Serve with a healthy dressing like the ones on pages 202–203.

Makes 1 serving

Low-Fat French Vinaigrette

INGREDIENTS

2 Tbsp	canola or safflower oil
⅓ cup	red wine vinegar
⅓ cup	fresh lemon juice
2 tsp	chopped fresh garlic
1 Tbsp	(heaping) Dijon mustard
1 Tbsp	orange juice
2 Tbsp	paprika
1 tsp	salt
½ tsp	ground pepper

DIRECTIONS

Add ingredients to a jar. Close lid tight.

Shake until mixed.

Makes 4–6 servings

Low-Fat Italian Dressing

⅓ cup	red wine vinegar
2 Tbsp	extra-virgin olive oil
¼ cup	fresh lemon juice
1 Tbsp	Dijon mustard
	Salt and pepper, to taste

DIRECTIONS

Add ingredients to a jar. Close lid tight.

Shake until mixed.

Makes 4–6 servings

Fruit and Vegetable Protein Boost

INGREDIENTS

8–12 oz	water, skim milk, or unsweetened almond milk
2	handfuls of ice cubes
1 scoop	100% whey protein
½ cup	berries of choice
½ cup	another fruit of choice, except banana (optional)
½ cup	chopped carrots
1 cup	fresh spinach
2 Tbsp	PB2 (optional)

DIRECTIONS

Add ingredients to a blender.

Blend until smooth.

Makes 1 serving

Banana Milkshake

INGREDIENTS

8–12 oz	water, skim milk, or unsweetened almond milk
2	handfuls of ice cubes
1 tsp	vanilla extract
1	whole banana
1	scoop 100% whey protein
1 Tbsp	PB2 (optional)

DIRECTIONS

Add ingredients to a blender.

Blend until smooth.

Makes 1 serving

Berries and Cream

INGREDIENTS

½ tsp	vanilla extract
¼ cup	low-fat ricotta cheese
2 tsp	fresh lemon juice
1 cup	mixed berries

DIRECTIONS

Mix together vanilla, ricotta cheese, and lemon juice in a bowl.

Top with berries.

Makes 1 serving

Berries and Cream
With Oranges and Fresh Mint

INGREDIENTS

1 cup	nonfat plain Greek yogurt
½ tsp	vanilla extract
¾ cup	berries of choice
1	orange, peeled and sliced
4	fresh mint leaves, chopped

DIRECTIONS

Mix together Greek yogurt and vanilla in a bowl.

Top with berries and orange slices.

Sprinkle on mint leaves.

Makes 1 serving

The Becoming Ageless Workout Plan

Your 12-week guide to being stronger and fitter eases you into training in the gym three days a week.

PROGRESS AT YOUR own comfortable pace. Remember that you're looking to develop a system that you believe is sustainable to follow for years, not weeks or months. If you can stick with it for 90 days, keeping it up afterward will, hopefully, become automatic.

As you progress and feel ready to hit the gym, consider working up to training your entire body up to three days a week. This total-body training strategy, according to research published in the *Journal of Strength and Conditioning Research*, is a more effective approach in regard to adding muscle compared with focusing on specific body parts. (In the study, the strength gains of the three-day-per-week total-body group were equal to those of the body-part-specific group.) Plus, diversifying your exercise selection exposes you to more exercises more often than a traditional body-part split does, which means you get more practice to iron out any form issues.

Eventually, you'll want to get into the habit of changing things up every three weeks or so—from equipment used to sets and reps completed to loads used. Doing so presents continual challenges to the muscles and central nervous system; failing to do so will lead to stagnation. For now, it's nothing to be concerned with.

Use the Becoming Ageless Workout Plan as a guide, but alter it as you see fit to progress safely and without injury. Spend at least four to 10 minutes warming up or cooling down with a dynamic stretch before and after each workout. Rest as needed between exercises and sets but aim to keep each session intense. For cardio, consider running, swimming, rowing, cycling, jumping rope, or any activity that gets your heart rate up. For a greater cardiovascular challenge, alternate periods of high intensity with a steady pace. As the weeks pass you'll work up to spending about an hour exercising per day. Refer to pages 222–237 for a full list of exercise descriptions.

The *Becoming Ageless* 12-Week Workout Plan

Week 1

Body-Weight Routine:
Do 5–10 reps of each exercise.

Cardio:
Walk.

Stretching Routine:
See page 61.

Day 1
Body-Weight Routine:
- Push-up
- Sit-up
- Air Squat

Day 2
Cardio:
10 minutes
- Steady-state

Day 3
Rest or Stretching Routine:
4–8 minutes

Week 2

Body-Weight Routine:
Do 5–10 reps for each exercise. Aim to complete 2–3 rounds if you feel up to it.

Cardio:
Walk or light jog.

Stretching Routine:
See page 61.

Day 1
Body-Weight Routine:
- Push-up
- Sit-up
- Air Squat

Day 2
Cardio:
10 minutes
- Steady-state

Stretching Routine:
4–8 minutes

Day 3
Body-Weight Routine:
- Push-up
- Sit-up
- Air Squat

*ROUND: Move from one exercise to the next until all exercises are completed.
SET: How many times you complete a given number of reps of an exercise.

Day 4

Body-Weight Routine:

- Push-up
- Sit-up
- Air Squat

Day 5

Cardio:
15 minutes

- Steady-state

Day 6

Stretching Routine:
4–8 minutes

Day 7

Rest or Cardio:
15 minutes

- Steady-state

Day 4

Rest or Cardio:
15 minutes

- Steady-state

Day 5

Body-Weight Routine:

- Push-up
- Sit-up
- Air Squat
- Burpee

Day 6

Rest or Cardio:
15 minutes

- Steady-state

Stretching Routine:
4–8 minutes

Day 7

***Cardio:**
20 minutes

- Steady-state

*Or substitute with a yoga class or a full-body stretching routine.

Week 3

Body-Weight Routine:
Do 5–10 reps of each exercise; try to cap your rest at 1 minute between moves. Attempt to complete 1 more round than you did the previous week.

Strength Circuit:
Complete 1 round of 5–10 reps per exercise.

Core Workout:
Perform as directed.

Cardio:
Jog, run, cycle, swim, row, use an elliptical machine, jump rope, or do any activity that increases your heart rate.

Stretching Routine:
See page 61.

Day 1

Body-Weight Routine:
- Push-up
- Sit-up
- Air Squat
- Burpee

Stretching Routine:
4–8 minutes

Day 2

Cardio:
25 minutes
- Steady-state

Day 3

Strength Circuit:
- Bench Press
- Deadlift
- Pull-up
- Dumbbell Squat
- Dumbbell Overhead Press
- Dumbbell Lunge
- Dumbbell Shrug
- Dumbbell Lateral Raise
- Dumbbell Curl

Day 4

Rest or Cardio:
15 minutes

- Steady-state

Day 5

Strength Circuit:

- Push-up
- Sit-up
- Air Squat

Core Workout:

- Plank 1 x 30 seconds
- Bicycle 2 x 10–15/side
- Russian Twist 1 x 10–15/side
- Leg Raise 2 x 10–15

Day 6

Rest or Cardio:
30 minutes

- HIIT for 3 minutes
- Steady-state for 15 minutes
- HIIT for 2 minutes
- Steady-state for 10 minutes

Day 7

*Cardio:
30 minutes

- Steady-state for 15 minutes
- HIIT for 2–3 minutes
- Steady-state for the duration

*Or substitute with a yoga class or a full-body stretching routine.

Week 4

Body-Weight Routine:
Do 5–10 reps of each exercise; cap your rest at 45 seconds between moves. Attempt to complete 1–2 more rounds than you did the previous week.

Strength Circuit:
Complete 1 round of 5–10 reps per exercise.

Core Workout:
Perform as directed.

Cardio:
Jog, run, cycle, swim, row, use an elliptical machine, jump rope, or do any activity that increases your heart rate.

Stretching Routine:
See page 61.

Day 1

Strength Circuit:
- Bench Press
- Deadlift
- Pull-up
- Dumbbell Squat
- Dumbbell Overhead Press
- Dumbbell Lunge
- Dumbbell Shrug
- Dumbbell Lateral Raise
- Dumbbell Curl
- Triceps Rope Pushdown

Day 2

*Cardio:
30 minutes
- Steady-state for 10 minutes
- HIIT for 2 minutes
- Steady-state for 10 minutes
- HIIT for 2 minutes
- Steady-state for the duration

Day 3

Body-Weight Routine:
- Push-up
- Sit-up
- Air Squat

Core Workout:
- Plank 1 x 30 seconds
- Bicycle 2 x 10–15/side
- Russian Twist 1 x 10–15/side
- Leg Raise 2 x 10–15

Day 4	Day 5	Day 6	Day 7
Rest or Cardio: 20 minutes	**Strength Circuit:**	**Cardio:** 20–30 minutes	**Rest or Cardio:** 10–15 minutes
■ Steady-state	■ Bench Press	■ Steady-state for 10 minutes	■ Steady-state
	■ Deadlift	■ HIIT for 2 minutes	
	■ Pull-up	■ Steady-state for 10 minutes	
	■ Dumbbell Squat	■ HIIT for 2 minutes	
	■ Dumbbell Overhead Press	■ Steady-state for the duration	
	■ Dumbbell Lunge		
	■ Dumbbell Shrug	**Stretching Routine:** 8–10 minutes	
	■ Dumbbell Lateral Raise		
	■ Barbell Curl		
	■ Triceps Rope Pushdown		

*Or substitute with a yoga class or a full-body stretching routine.

Strength Circuit:
Complete 2 rounds of 8–12 reps per exercise.

Core Workout:
Perform as directed.

Cardio:
Jog, run, cycle, swim, row, use an elliptical machine, jump rope, or do any activity that increases your heart rate.

Stretching Routine:
See page 61.

Day 1

Strength Circuit:

- Barbell Squat
- Incline Bench Press
- Lat Pulldown
- Kettlebell Romanian Deadlift
- Barbell Overhead Press
- Dumbbell Step-up
- Barbell Shrug
- Bentover Lateral Raise
- Dumbbell Hammer Curl
- Seated Overhead Triceps Extension

Day 2

*Cardio:
20 minutes

- Steady-state for 8 minutes
- HIIT for 3 minutes
- Steady-state for 7 minutes
- HIIT for the duration

Day 3

Strength Circuit:

- Barbell Squat
- Incline Bench Press
- Lat Pulldown
- Kettlebell Romanian Deadlift
- Barbell Overhead Press
- Dumbbell Step-up
- Barbell Shrug
- Bentover Lateral Raise
- Hammer Curl
- Seated Overhead Triceps Extension

Core Workout:

- Plank 1 x 30 seconds
- Bicycle 2 x 10–25/side
- Russian Twist 1 x 10–25/side
- Leg Raise 2 x 10–25

Day 4

Rest or *Cardio:
15 minutes

- Steady-state

Day 5

Strength Circuit:

- Barbell Squat
- Incline Bench Press
- Lat Pulldown
- Kettlebell Romanian Deadlift
- Barbell Overhead Press
- Dumbbell Step-up
- Barbell Shrug
- Bentover Lateral Raise
- Dumbbell Hammer Curl
- Seated Overhead Triceps Extension

Core Workout:

- Plank 1 x 30 seconds
- Bicycle 2 x 10–25/side
- Russian Twist 1 x 10–25/side
- Leg Raise 2 x 10–25

Day 6

Cardio:
8–10 minutes

- HIIT for 2–4 minutes
- Steady-state for 3 minutes
- HIIT for the duration

Day 7

Rest or Cardio:
15 minutes

- HIIT for 3 minutes
- Steady-state for the duration

Stretching Routine:
8–10 minutes

*Or substitute with a yoga class or a full-body stretching routine.

Weeks 6-7

Strength Circuit:
Complete 2–3 rounds of 8–12 reps per exercise on Day 1 and Day 5. On Day 3, use a slightly heavier weight than used on Day 1 and complete 5 reps for each exercise.

Core Workout:
Perform as directed.

Cardio:
Jog, run, cycle, swim, row, use an elliptical machine, jump rope, or do any activity that increases your heart rate.

Stretching Routine:
See page 61.

Week 8

Strength Circuit:
Complete 3 rounds of 8–12 reps per exercise.

Core Workout:
Perform as directed.

Cardio:
Jog, run, cycle, swim, row, use an elliptical machine, jump rope, or do any activity that increases your heart rate.

Stretching Routine:
See page 61.

Day 1

Strength Circuit:

■ Barbell Squat

■ Incline Bench Press

■ Lat Pulldown

■ Kettlebell Romanian Deadlift

■ Barbell Overhead Press

■ Dumbbell Step-up

■ Barbell Shrug

■ Bentover Lateral Raise

■ Dumbbell Hammer Curl

■ Seated Overhead Triceps Extension

Core Workout:

■ Plank 1 x 30 seconds

■ Bicycle 2 x 15–20/side

■ Russian Twist 1 x 15–20/side

■ Leg Raise 2 x 15–20

Day 2

*Cardio:
30 minutes

■ Steady-state for 20 minutes

■ HIIT for 4–5 minutes

■ Steady-state for the duration

Day 3

Strength Circuit:

- Barbell Squat
- Bench Press
- Pull-up
- Kettlebell Romanian Deadlift
- Barbell Overhead Press
- Dumbbell Step-up
- Barbell Shrug
- Bentover Lateral Raise
- Dumbbell Curl
- Seated Overhead Triceps Extension

Day 4

Rest or Cardio: 20 minutes

- Steady-state

Day 5

Strength Circuit:

- Barbell Squat
- Incline Bench Press
- Lat Pulldown
- Deadlift
- Barbell Overhead Press
- Dumbbell Step-up
- Barbell Shrug
- Bentover Lateral Raise
- Dumbbell Hammer Curl
- Seated Overhead Triceps Extension

Core Workout:

- Plank 1 x 30 seconds
- Bicycle 2 x 15–20/side
- Russian Twist 1 x 15–20/side
- Leg Raise 2 x 15–20

Day 6

Rest or Cardio: 12–15 minutes

- HIIT for 4–6 minutes
- Steady-state for the duration

Day 7

Cardio: 15 minutes

- Steady-state for 5 minutes
- HIIT for 4–5 minutes
- Steady-state for the duration

*Or substitute with a yoga class or a full-body stretching routine.

Weeks 9–10

Strength Routine:
On Days 1 and 7, complete 3 sets of 8–12 reps per exercise before moving on to the next move. Rest about 30 seconds between sets. On Day 3, complete 3 sets of 5 reps per exercise using a slightly heavier weight than you used on Day 1.

Core Workout:
Perform as directed.

Cardio:
Jog, run, cycle, swim, row, use an elliptical machine, jump rope, or do any activity that increases your heart rate.

Stretching Routine:
See page 61.

Week 11

Strength Routine:
On Days 1 and 7, complete 3 sets of 5 reps per exercise. On Day 3, complete 3 sets of 8–12 reps per exercise.

Core Workout:
Perform as directed.

Cardio:
Jog, run, cycle, swim, row, use an elliptical machine, jump rope, or do any activity that increases your heart rate.

Stretching Routine:
See page 61.

Week 12

Strength Routine:
On Days 1 and 3, complete 3 sets of 12 reps per exercise. On Day 7, complete 3–5 sets of 5 reps per exercise.

Core Workout:
Perform as directed.

Cardio:
Jog, run, cycle, swim, row, use an elliptical machine, jump rope, or do any activity that increases your heart rate.

Stretching Routine:
See page 61.

Day 1

Strength Routine:
- Barbell Squat
- Bench Press
- Lat Pulldown
- Kettlebell Romanian Deadlift
- Barbell Overhead Press
- Dumbbell Step-up
- Barbell Shrug
- Bentover Lateral Raise
- Barbell Curl
- Seated Overhead Triceps Extension

Core Workout:
- Plank 1 x 30 seconds
- Bicycle 2 x 15–20/side
- Russian Twist 1 x 15–20/side
- Leg Raise 2 x 15–20

After completing Week 12, shake up your routine: Change exercises, set/rep schemes, rest times, and volume.

Day 2

*Cardio:
20–30 minutes

- Steady-state for 10 minutes
- HIIT for 3 minutes
- Steady-state for 3 minutes
- HIIT for 3 minutes
- Steady-state for the duration

Day 3

Strength Routine:

- Barbell Squat
- Bench Press
- Lat Pulldown
- Kettlebell Romanian Deadlift
- Barbell Overhead Press
- Dumbbell Step-up
- Barbell Shrug
- Bentover Lateral Raise
- Dumbbell Curl
- Seated Overhead Triceps Extension

Core Workout:

- Plank 1 x 30 seconds
- Bicycle 2 x 15–20/side
- Russian Twist 1 x 15–20/side
- Leg Raise 2 x 15–20

Day 4

Rest or Cardio:
20–30 minutes

- Steady-state for 10 minutes
- HIIT for 3 minutes
- Steady-state for 3 minutes
- HIIT for 3 minutes
- Steady-state for the duration

Day 5

Cardio:
15–20 minutes

- Steady-state for 5 minutes
- HIIT for 2 minutes
- Steady-state for 5 minutes
- HIIT for 2 minutes
- Steady-state for the duration

Day 6

Rest or Cardio:
12–15 minutes

- HIIT for 8–10 minutes
- Steady-state for the duration

Day 7

Strength Routine:

- Barbell Squat
- Incline Bench Press
- Pull-up
- Kettlebell Romanian Deadlift
- Barbell Overhead Press
- Dumbbell Step-up
- Barbell Shrug
- Bentover Lateral Raise
- Dumbbell Curl
- Seated Overhead Triceps Extension

Core Workout:

- Plank 1 x 30 seconds
- Bicycle 2 x 15–20/side
- Russian Twist 1 x 15–20/side
- Leg Raise 2 x 15–20

*Or substitute with a yoga class or a full-body stretching routine.

THESE PRIMARILY TARGET the MUSCLES in the CHEST, BACK, and LEGS.

BENCH PRESS

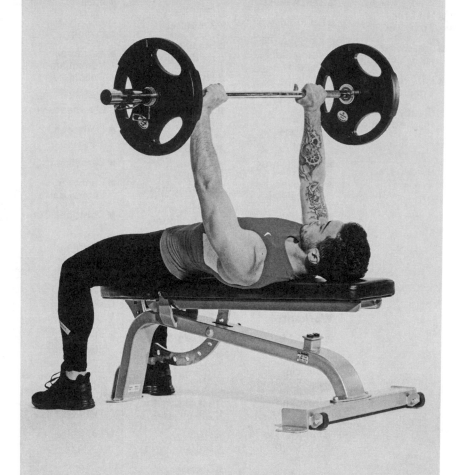

L ie on a bench and grasp the bar at shoulder width. Lift the bar off the rack and, keeping your elbows close to your body, lower the bar to just above your chest, and then press it back up. Use a spotter.

INCLINE
BENCH PRESS

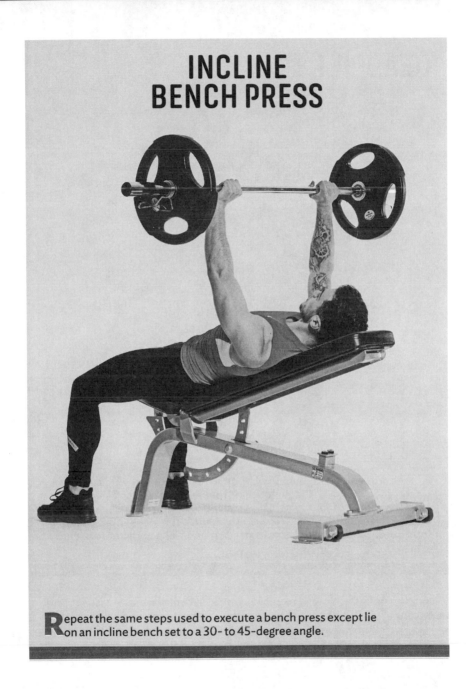

Repeat the same steps used to execute a bench press except lie on an incline bench set to a 30- to 45-degree angle.

DEADLIFT

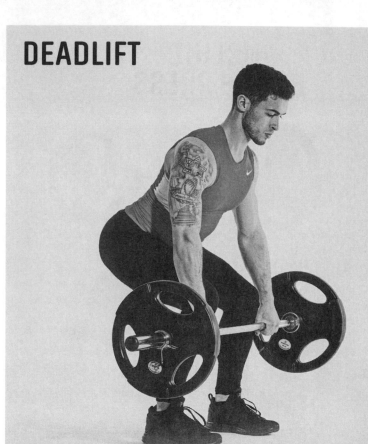

Stand with your feet shoulder-width apart and hold a barbell just outside shoulder width with the bar touching your shins. (Your hands should be on the outside of your shins, palms facing back.) Keeping a slight bend in your knees, bend at your waist until the barbell is a few inches off the floor; arch your back, keep your chest and head up, and stand upright. Do not round your back.

Kettlebell Romanian Deadlift
Hold a pair of kettlebells in front of your waist. Slightly bend your knees and shift your hips back. Keep your chest up as you lower the kettlebell toward the floor. Go as low as you can without rounding your back, and squeeze through your hamstrings and glutes as you slowly return to the start position.

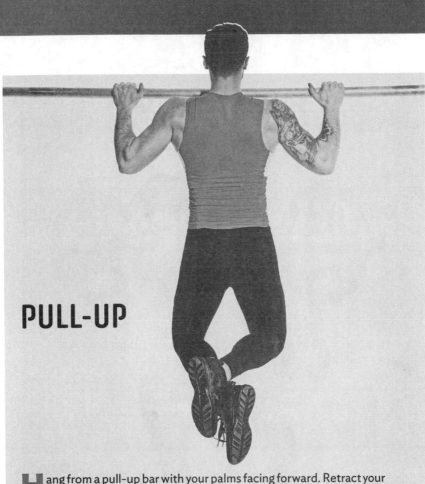

PULL-UP

Hang from a pull-up bar with your palms facing forward. Retract your shoulder blades to focus on the lats and rhomboids and pull yourself up until your chin rises above the bar. Then slowly lower yourself to a dead-hang position (with arms completely straight). If you're unable to complete a pull-up with strict form—you can't lower yourself all the way down and pull yourself up so your chin is above the bar—ask a spotter to assist you. If you are alone, wrap an elastic exercise band around the bar, place a foot or a knee in the hanging loop, and use the tension in the band to assist you. Alternatively, you can do machine-assisted pull-ups or lat pulldowns on a weight-stack machine.

Lat Pulldown
Sit at a lat pulldown station and grasp the bar outside *shoulder width. Focus on pulling with your lats, not your biceps, as you bring the* *bar to your collarbone or upper chest and drive your elbows back and down.*

BARBELL SQUAT

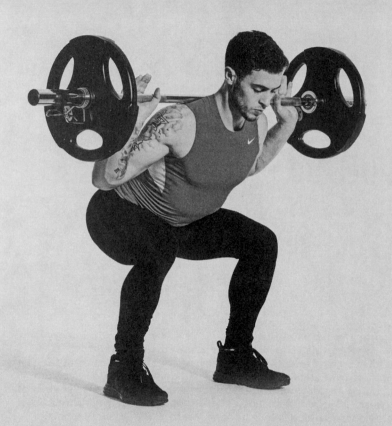

Stand with feet shoulder-width apart and your toes pointed out slightly with a loaded barbell resting along your upper traps. Grasp the bar wider than shoulder width and stand, keeping your toes pointed slightly outward. Breathe in, bend at the hips, and bend your knees to lower your body as far as you can without compromising the arch in your lower back. Aim to descend until your thighs are parallel with the floor. Then explode back up and squeeze your glutes and core at the top.

DUMBBELL SQUAT

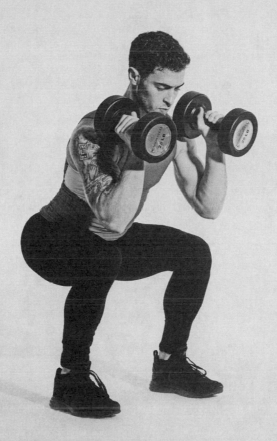

Stand holding two dumbbells at shoulder level. Sit your butt back and bend your legs to lower yourself into a squat position as low as possible or until your legs are just below parallel with the floor. Feel the weight in your heels, not your toes. Keep your chest up and your back straight. Press your feet into the floor to rise to the standing position and repeat.

THESE WILL HELP YOU BUILD UPPER- and LOWER-BODY STRENGTH and SUPPORT YOUR MAIN LIFTS.

DUMBBELL LUNGE

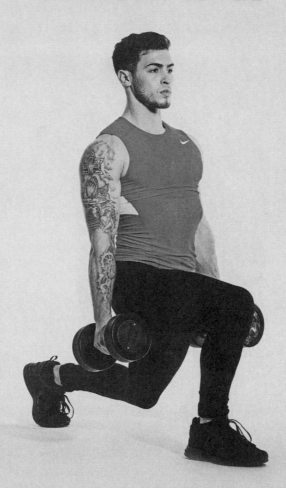

Hold a pair of dumbbells at your side. Step forward so that your front leg forms a right angle and your back knee nearly touches the floor. Be sure that your front knee does not extend past your toes. Push with your forward heel to stand back up, then lunge forward with your opposite foot. Continue alternating this way for the prescribed repetitions.

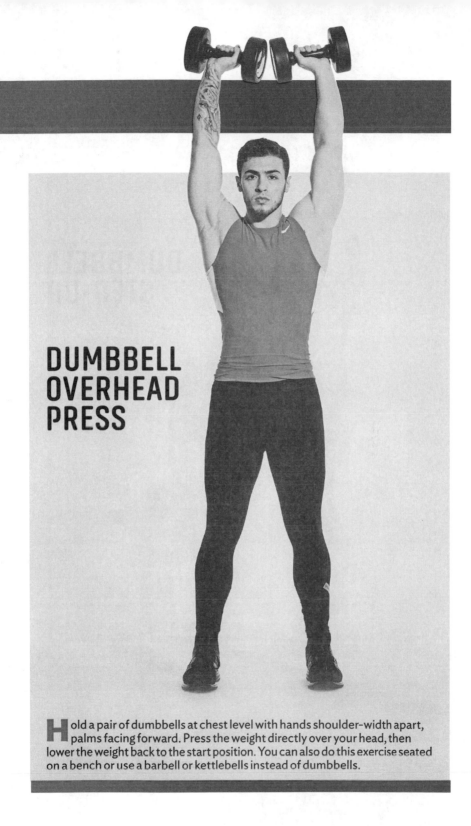

DUMBBELL OVERHEAD PRESS

Hold a pair of dumbbells at chest level with hands shoulder-width apart, palms facing forward. Press the weight directly over your head, then lower the weight back to the start position. You can also do this exercise seated on a bench or use a barbell or kettlebells instead of dumbbells.

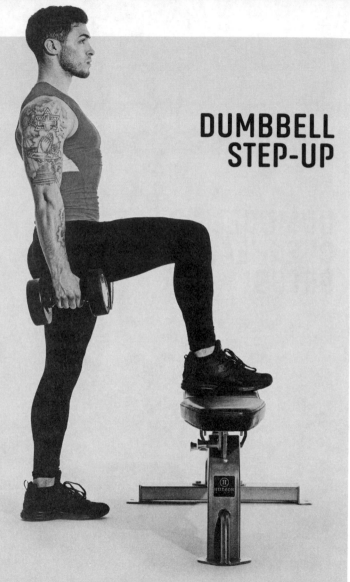

DUMBBELL STEP-UP

Stand in front of a bench or box while holding a dumbbell in each hand. Keep one leg straight, place one foot on the bench, and then stand up on the bench. Do not use your grounded leg to execute the lift. Once both feet are on the bench or box, step down and repeat.

Dumbbell Shrug
Grasp a pair of dumbbells and hold them by your sides, palms facing your legs. Without using momentum or bending your arms, attempt to lift your shoulders to your ears. Pause at the top, then slowly lower the weights to the start position. You can also use a barbell or kettlebells.

Dumbbell Lateral Raise
Hold a pair of light dumbbells at your sides, palms facing in. Keeping your arms straight, raise your arms outward to shoulder level, then lower and repeat.

Triceps Rope Pushdown
Grasp a rope attachment that's fixed to a high-pulley cable. Pull the weight down until your arms are slightly above a 90-degree angle and push the weight down until your arms are straight. Flare to about shoulder width at the bottom of the movement. Allow the weight to return to about the right-angle position and repeat.

Bentover Lateral Raise
Hold a dumbbell in each hand, palms facing each other, and bend over until your upper body is nearly parallel to the floor. Aim to keep your lower back flat as you raise the weights out 90 degrees, and then squeeze your shoulder blades together at the move's apex.

Dumbbell Curl
Hold a pair of dumbbells at your sides, palms facing forward. Keep your elbows tight to your body and curl the weight toward your shoulders. Lower the weights slowly. You can also use a barbell. If you find that this exercise hurts your wrists, perform it using a neutral or hammer grip.

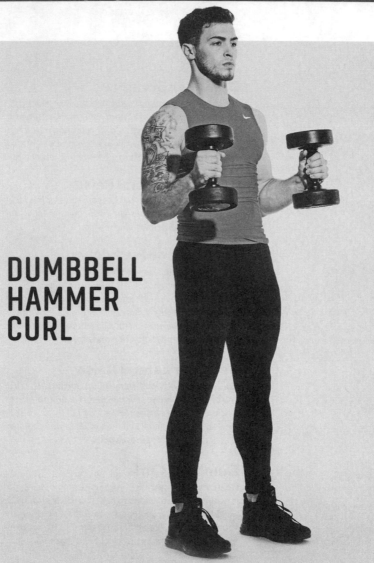

DUMBBELL HAMMER CURL

Hold a dumbbell in each hand at your sides. (Your palms should face your body.) Keep your upper arms against your sides as you bring the weight up, allowing your elbows to travel slightly in front of your body. Pause at the top, then return to the start position. Alternate arms or curl the weights at the same time.

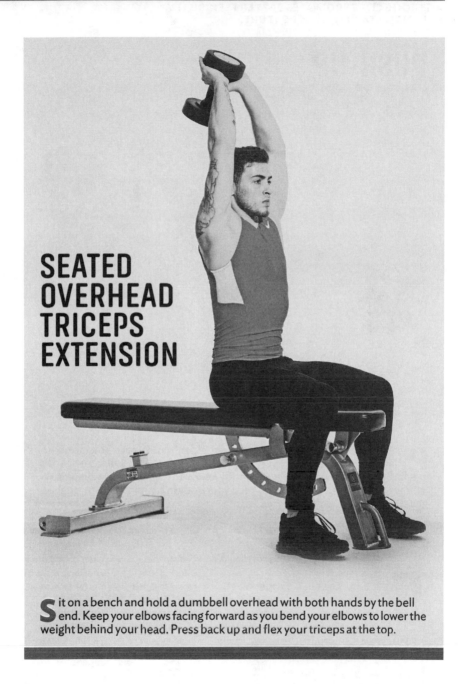

SEATED OVERHEAD TRICEPS EXTENSION

Sit on a bench and hold a dumbbell overhead with both hands by the bell end. Keep your elbows facing forward as you bend your elbows to lower the weight behind your head. Press back up and flex your triceps at the top.

A STRONG CORE PROMOTES BETTER FLEXIBILITY, BALANCE, STABILITY, and POSTURE.

PUSH-UP

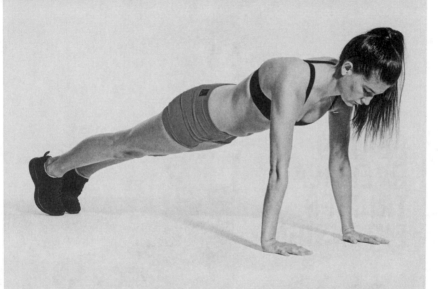

Place your hands on the floor roughly shoulder-width apart. Your arms should be straight, and your back should form a straight line from head to heels. Bend your arms to lower your body nearly to the floor while keeping your elbows close to your body. Aim to keep your body in a straight line throughout the movement. (Don't allow your hips to sag.)

Bicycle

Lie faceup, interlace your fingertips behind your head, and pull your bent knees to your chest, contracting your abs. Lift your shoulder blades off the floor, but don't bend or pull your neck forward. Now straighten your right leg and rotate your upper body to the left, bringing your right elbow to touch your left knee. Next, straighten your left leg while bringing your right knee to your chest and rotating your torso to touch that knee with your left elbow. Continue alternating this way for the prescribed reps per side.

PLANK

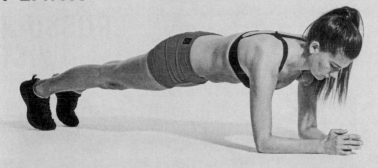

Get into push-up position, bend your elbows, and rest your weight on your forearms. Brace your abs and maintain a flat back from head to heels. Try to hold this position for 30 seconds without allowing your hips to sag. Gradually work your way up to a 60-second hold.

LEG RAISE

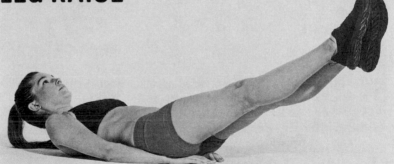

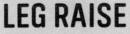

Lie on your back with your hands at your sides, palms touching the floor near your glutes. Keep your legs straight as you lift them 6 to 12 inches off the floor. Hold for a second, then lower. That's 1 rep.

BUILD LEAN MUSCLE, IMPROVE FLEXIBILITY, and GIVE YOUR METABOLISM a BOOST USING JUST YOUR OWN BODY WEIGHT.

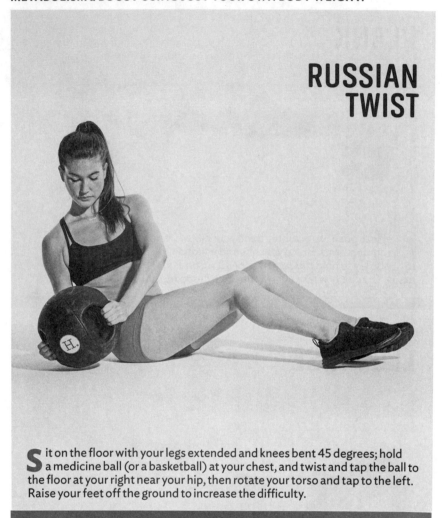

RUSSIAN TWIST

Sit on the floor with your legs extended and knees bent 45 degrees; hold a medicine ball (or a basketball) at your chest, and twist and tap the ball to the floor at your right near your hip, then rotate your torso and tap to the left. Raise your feet off the ground to increase the difficulty.

Air Squat

With your feet shoulder-width apart and pointing out slightly, take a deep breath, push your hips back, and bend your knees as if sitting into a chair. Keep your chest up and do not round your back. Squat down until your thighs are lower than parallel to the floor, if possible. As you become stronger, add resistance by using kettle-bells, dumbbells, or a barbell.

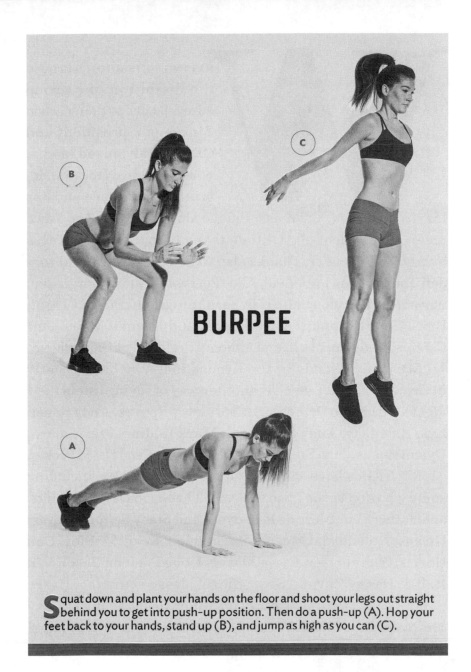

BURPEE

S quat down and plant your hands on the floor and shoot your legs out straight behind you to get into push-up position. Then do a push-up (A). Hop your feet back to your hands, stand up (B), and jump as high as you can (C).

Acknowledgments

WRITING THIS BOOK has been the definition of a group effort. I'd like to thank David Zinczenko, president and CEO of Galvanized Media, who encouraged me to write it in the first place and has inspired, cajoled, and reassured me along the way. And I owe an enormous debt of gratitude to my co-author and fitness buddy, Zack Zeigler. Thanks also to Ted Spiker; copy editors Jeff Tomko, Yeun Littlefield, Alice Perry, and Muriel Jorgensen; our able researcher, April Hines; photographers Brad Trent, Erica Schultz, and Marius Bugge; and Keenan Mayo, Jeff Csatari, Andy Turnbull, and Michael Freidson of Galvanized.

My many friends in the fitness industry have greatly informed this text (which is another way of saying I stole their ideas). Thanks to Dr. Peter Attia, Harvey Spevak, Andy Speer, Eric Rakofsky, Andy Slizewski, Mark Rodino, Flex Cabral, Dyan Tsiumis, Julia Stephens, JH McNierney, and David Pecker.

My friends have encouraged me along the way, including some who don't even train with me. Thanks to David Remnick and Esther Fein, Marc de la Bruyere and Stacy Schiff, Andrew Farkas, Roland and Maggie Hernandez, Kevin Dorsey, Dan Harris, Sam Houser, Steve Marks, Doug Polaner, Jason Van Itallie, Danny Zevnik, Scott Siegel, Jesse Dufresne, Harry Santa-Olalla, Jeb Gaybrick, Zach Miller, Josh Kushner, Ricky Van Veen and Allison Williams, Justin Shaffer and Annabel Teal, Sam Lessin, Jay Hass, Paul Viera, Willy Walker, Ron

Beller, Kevin Ryan, Paddy Walker, Erik Eason, Richie Cornell, John Bradshaw, Greg Tanenbaum, Kelly McGarrity, Brent Craft, Billy Raiford, Robert and Tracey Pruzan, Tony and Shelly Malkin, William Lauder, Matthew Bronfman, Barry Sternlicht, Rick Rubens, Michael Dornemann, J Moses, Josh Felser, Wade Davis, and Michael Sheresky. And thanks also to my mentors Dick Parsons, Don Godel, and Barry Diller, who keep me searching for excellence.

Thanks, too, to my assistants, Maya Bronfman, Teo Varga, and Katerina Benitez, and my friends and colleagues at ZMC and Take-Two: Jordan Turkewitz, Andrew Vogel, Seymour Sammell, Karl Slatoff, Brian Motechin, Jason Sporer, Ripan Kadakia, Sheila Dharmarajan, Beau Duncan, Ben Carus, Jenn Kolbe, Scott Lucas, Spencer Kushner, Lainie Goldstein, Hank Diamond, Alan Lewis, Chris Casazza, Michael Worosz, and Dan Emerson.

I want to thank everyone who participates in The Program, especially Scott Hernandez, James Green, and Nick Sizer for making it happen in the first place, and more recently the entire leadership crew, especially Ryan Nowack, Tony Richardson, and Eric Posner.

Most important, I want to thank my three beautiful and talented and always-obedient children, Cooper, Lucas, and Leigh, and my incredibly patient wife, Wendy, who really, really doesn't like me getting up at 5 a.m.

Strauss Zelnick

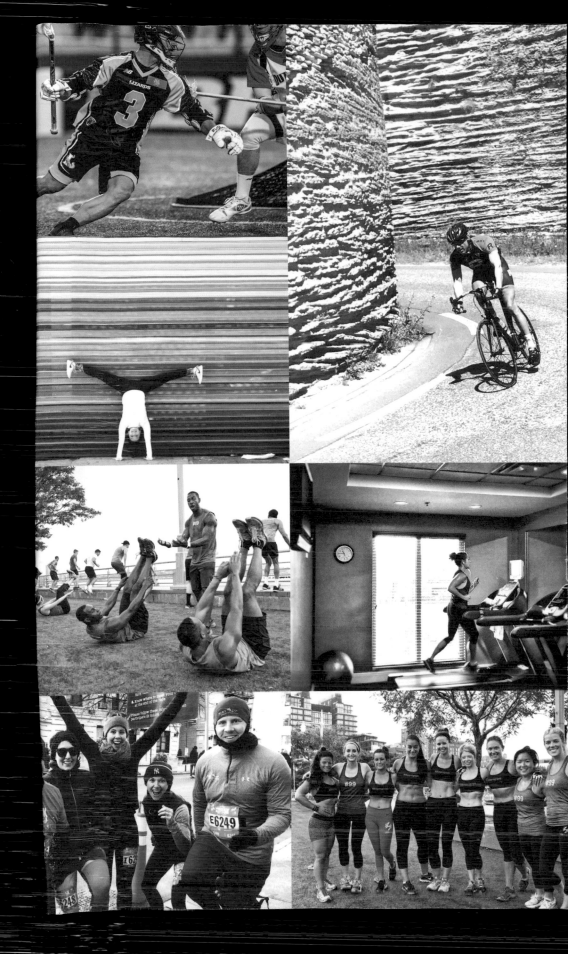

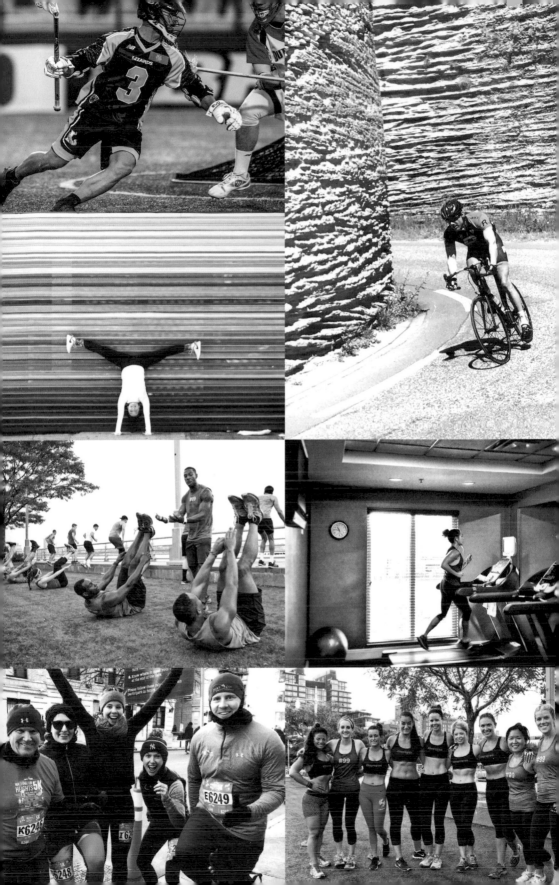